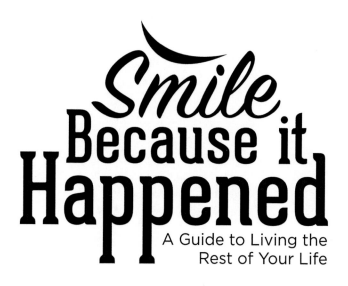

Smile
Because it
Happened

A Guide to Living the
Rest of Your Life

Carole Young *&* Stacey Reynolds

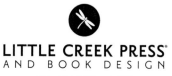

LITTLE CREEK PRESS
AND BOOK DESIGN

Mineral Point, Wisconsin USA

Little Creek Press®
A Division of Kristin Mitchell Design, Inc.
5341 Sunny Ridge Road
Mineral Point, Wisconsin 53565

Book Design and Project Coordination:
Little Creek Press

First Edition
August 2019

Printed in Wisconsin, United States of America

To order books visit www.littlecreekpress.com

Library of Congress Control Number: 2019909516

ISBN-13: 978-1-942586-61-6

On the front cover:
Stacey on the deck of Red Oak cabin, Fay Lake, Long Lake, WI, 2008

For Aleksander, Kassia and Jakoby

Thank you to Tommy for allowing this book to happen and
to my family members who were always positive and encouraging.
Thank you to Little Creek Press' Kristin Mitchell and editors
Diane Franklin and Shannon Booth for guiding me
through the process which resulted in this beautiful
book, a wonderful testament to Stacey.

Table of Contents

... still, some people blaze through life like comets, leaving incredibly bright, but tragically short, displays of light that we can only wonder why so many beautiful things are so temporary.

I can imagine someone in the Great Beyond, pointing to the map of her life, and saying, "You see that? That is how to live life on Earth."

Mark Steel

CHAPTER 1

Seattle, Here We Come!

Carole

"I have something to tell you." Daughter Stacey sequestered me in a corner of her grandmother's dining room. "I want to tell you before you hear it from somebody else." It was Easter Sunday, 1995. She and husband Tommy had come from Milwaukee to celebrate the day with family members. My thoughts at that moment were, "I'm going to be a grandma! My first grandbaby!" But the news was that she and Tommy were leaving Wisconsin and moving to Washington State—Seattle. It seemed so far away! About as far as you can go and still be in the United States. All four of my children had always lived within a few hours' drive. It wasn't the happy news I was hoping for.

They packed their belongings in a rental truck, towing their car with pet cats Mosely and Creepy inside, and began their cross-country adventure in the summer of 1995 without the convenience of GPS or cell phones. Upon arriving in Seattle, Stacey would keep her interior design job with a Fond du Lac, Wisconsin, company that specialized in themed McDonald's, opening up a western branch, and Tommy would be employed in the IT industry.

After renting an apartment for a short time, they purchased a condo, and when more room was needed to accommodate their growing family, they rented out the condo and moved to a rental home in the Wallingford district of Seattle.

Letter postmarked July 19, 1995, from 121 Vine St., #303, Seattle, Washington

We have now been in Seattle for two full weeks. It's time I sat down and documented some of our adventures moving to the "jet city."

First of all, if anyone ever tells you they are going to pack up all their belongings, drive 2,000 miles, end up in the downtown of a large city, and unload a 15-foot truck with only two people, tell them they're crazy. We pulled out of Milwaukee at about 8:30 p.m. on a Saturday night, which was about 12 hours later than we had wanted to start the trip. But the short drive and overnight stay in Madison was 90 miles off our long haul to Sioux Falls the next day, and we got to have breakfast with my sister, Lesley, that morning, which was an added bonus.

DAY ONE

We left Madison refreshed and rested but still a little zombie-like. We stopped for lunch and to switch drivers in Albert Lea, Minnesota. The truck stop had a strange windmill theme. I paid special attention to the wooden shoes attached to the pendant lamps. Perhaps this might be something I could use in a McDonald's that really wanted to "go nuts." I had cottage cheese and iceberg lettuce, which would be my truck stop staple for a few days. It was difficult to be a vegetarian or a healthy eater of any type for that matter on this trip. After we were all refueled, we went back out to the truck. Before taking off, we checked on the cats in the car. Tommy checked on Creepy on the passenger side, and I checked on Mosely on the driver side. Mosely cried incessantly. There was a mental checklist of things we had to remember about driving, especially when it came down to keys and not locking ourselves out. We had to keep our only car key in the ignition of the car when in motion because the car had to be in neutral. We also had to remember not to lock the car doors when the key was in the ignition. Given the fact that we were both still mentally fatigued from the many days that led up to this move we weren't thinking about keys when we both slammed the car doors at the very same time. However, we were both sharp enough to realize what we did instantly. The cats were locked in the car in their carriers without a litter box! But we wouldn't be able to do anything about it for at least another 250 miles. For now, we would concentrate on our next adventure: Stacey behind the wheel of the big truck...

If you can picture me in somewhat of a cramped position with white knuckles and my head poked out so far over the steering wheel it is almost touching the window, then you have a pretty good picture of what my first 100 miles were like. I loosened up after a while. The road was straight and wide, and we were only 150 miles from our first destination. Our timing on this first day was not the best. We made many stops for food, for gas, to check the truck, and to use the bathroom, none of which seemed to happen at the same time; therefore, it was dark by the time we reached Sioux Falls. I had planned the trip carefully and had reservations for four Super 8 hotels across the country. Our special Super 8 VIP card gave us a discount of 10%. Other than that, our criteria for hotels was as follows: clean, cheap, nation-wide chain with toll-free reservations, and they take cats. No deluxe accommodations for these travelers.

I had called Super 8 to change all our reservations since we were one day behind the planned schedule. Based on past experience, I had confirmation numbers and addresses written down for all of the motels where we were going to stay... something every good traveler should have handy. These were etched out somewhat randomly on a sheet of paper. Maybe a little too randomly. As we approached Sioux Falls, in the dark, I asked Tommy to pull out the paper and tell me which exit to take. Exit 59, the Airport Super 8. That was odd, because we were now at exit 351. But the numbers were going down, so we decided to keep going. It was now very dark, raining quite hard, there was road construction, and we had no clue where we were going. I was tired and disoriented from driving, so my reflexes were slow, and I have trouble seeing at night. This was not fun. We went by signs for the airport, but there was no sign of exit 59. Tommy was upset because I was driving 40 miles per hour on the interstate. I was now in my cramped driving position again and claiming I couldn't see. Our first (and only) verbal confrontation of the trip ensued.

We got off at the next exit. After maneuvering through what seemed like an endless series of turns and stops, I pulled into a supermarket/ pizza parlor parking lot. I was totally stressed, and we both had to go to the bathroom really bad. Fortunately for us, we could use the facilities in the pizza parlor. Our cats weren't as lucky. They were still locked in the car and hadn't had a litter box in over five hours. I was in a trance-like state, so it's difficult to remember what happened when we asked the friendly people at the supermarket and pizza parlor for directions, but I do remember the people being somewhat vague (or was it us?). They had a difficult time telling us where we were or how to get back to Sioux Falls, and there was no phone we could use. We left the place very puzzled and shared a couple of jokes about the experience. This eased the tension that had built up between us and the worry about our cats. We stopped at a nearby gas station, where I called the motel and got clear directions. There was no exit 59. I wondered about this but was relieved we were only 10 miles past our destination, and Tommy had taken over the driving!

We found the motel without too much of a problem. This Super 8 was strategically placed next to a Happy Chef 24-hour restaurant (or was the restaurant strategically placed by it?) and, also, a sport's bar. We entered the motel check-in area and experienced a few moments of panic when the guy at the desk told us he had no reservation for us, but then relief when we found out it was in Tommy's name. I told him about our dilemma with the cats and finding the place. He recommended a locksmith and then began filling me in on how the interstate system works—north, south, east, west, numbers going down, numbers going up. My eyes glazed over. My mind was not ready for this unsolicited information. In the meantime, Tommy, the handyman, had taken the whole car apart and gotten into it. I didn't even care how he did it at that point. I just think he's pretty amazing sometimes.

Our motel room was about what we paid for—extremely small. I don't think we have ever stayed in a room so small. Well, maybe that old hotel in Vancouver. The headboard was no longer firmly attached to the wall or the bed for that matter. There must have been some ruckus going on in there before us. I didn't care to think about that! The cats loved it. They immediately warmed up to their surroundings. I guess anything was better than bouncing around in the back of a car slanted at a 15-degree angle for eight hours. We had to get out and stretch a bit (the room wasn't big enough for that) and decided after a day like today the sport's bar sounded better than deep fried food.

DAY TWO

It was probably about 9:00 when we woke up the next morning. We didn't have a clock, so we never really knew what time it was. This didn't seem to matter because on the road we were more tuned in to the miles to our next destination rather than the time of day. We were not aggressive about hitting the road at 6:00 a.m. or 8:00 a.m. or even 9:00 a.m. Our daily ritual began when we woke up, whenever that was. We showered and then went to Happy Chef for breakfast. There would be many more Happy Chefs in the days to come. This morning, I would have my first oatmeal, hash browns breakfast, and Tommy would have his first big cheesy omelet. We both indulged in some really bad coffee. After breakfast, we were totally refreshed. We went back to the room to check out and collect the cats. Creepy was under the covers of the bed. Mosely had crawled under the bed. I think they knew what their fate was. I was the morning shift driver. After our argument the night before, it was decided we would split all driving equally, and I had decided in my own head I would not be a wimp. I would drive the morning shift and deal with whatever weather or topography I might encounter on that shift.

The first thing we had to do was get gas. I pulled in to the next easy-on/easy-off stop on the interstate. This stop seemed to take forever since we both used the restroom, purchased beverages, and filled the tank with 33 gallons of diesel fuel. Tommy insisted I fill the tank this time. He thought I should learn this in case I ever need to do it again (in another life maybe). I went along with it since, after all, I was not a wimp. Once fueled up, we pulled out and were off on day two of our big adventure. A responsibility we had with the truck was to carefully document mileage at state lines and obtain gas receipts at all stops. This, of course, was the job of the passenger since the driver had enough on their mind. After driving about 10 minutes, I thought to ask Tommy if he had obtained the last receipt. He forgot. We calculated the potential penalty of this small oversight to be about $140. It was definitely worth it to go back. Day two got off to a somewhat rocky start.

If you've ever driven through South Dakota between Sioux Falls and Rapid City you know about the visual assault of billboards you encounter. Our first Wall Drug sign was at the Minnesota border just outside of LaCrosse, Wisconsin. After that, we saw them about every five miles. There was also Reptile Gardens and the man who carved Mount Rushmore, whose story was apparently more fascinating than the stone sculptures themselves, and, of course, the Mitchell Corn Palace. Every billboard provided you with some new and fascinating insight about what these tourist hotspots had to offer. I must admit I was drawn to these places more and more with every billboard. Not for what these places had to offer but for the kitsch appeal. I admire anyone who can drive through this state without being trapped.

The most thought-provoking billboards seemed to be of a fascist nature. "South Dakota rejects animal rights activists—livestock is our livelihood." This abrupt message did not make us vegetarians feel very welcome in the state.

In spite of the uncomfortable feelings some of these billboards conjured up, I was beginning to have some positive feelings and reflections about this trip. There wasn't much else to do but reflect and read billboards when driving through this part of South Dakota. I remembered the trip my family took out here. Could it be 20 years ago? I also compared our journey to those our ancestors took many years ago in covered wagons. This was a covered wagon of sorts.

We stopped in Mitchell because we had to see the World's Only Corn Palace. We parked the truck and walked a few blocks to see this architectural phenomenon. I remembered it as being much more fascinating when I was a kid. I think maybe it seemed like there was more corn then. Things always seem larger than life when you're a kid. We were a little disappointed but really glad to say we saw it. Before leaving town, we stopped at a miniature mall to get some food, any food. We were hungry. We were surprised to find a natural food store. "An oasis in the desert."

As we approached our next destination, Rapid City, the Wall Drug signs became more and more numerous, first every half mile, then every quarter mile, and then every 100 feet. We were trapped by the time we got to Wall, South Dakota. We were ready for that 5-cent cup of coffee and free water.

We arrived in Rapid City and found our motel without any problems. By now, we realized that exit 59 was for this stop and not Sioux Falls. I think it was also about this time we learned that the exit numbers correlated with the miles to the next state line. I think that was what the guy at the hotel was trying to tell me the night before.

Our hotel room was much better than the previous night. Tommy was in heaven because there was a reclining Lazy Boy chair and a remote control. It was a good thing because we were condemned to our room for the night. Motel rules: "Pets cannot be left unattended." Of course, we obeyed the rule since they had our $25 pet deposit. We ordered a pizza and went to bed.

DAY THREE

We must have felt a little more adventurous in the morning because we went to Happy Chef and left the cats alone. We decided the hash browns at this Happy Chef were a little better than yesterday. There were IQ test games on the tables of the restaurant. Tommy and I took turns cheating to see who could get the best score. When we returned to the room, we were surprised to find both cats had vanished. We eventually found Creepy under the covers, but where was Mosely? After searching every corner of the room, we found her inside the box spring of the bed. Apparently, they knew the routine now and were doing everything possible to avoid the inevitable.

After acquiring our cats and our $25 pet deposit, we were on our way out of the state. I started the driving again. I was much more comfortable with driving now, although I was slightly worried about the weather. (Of course, I didn't admit this because I wasn't a wimp.) The report the previous night said there was a winter storm warning in our travel path, 40-mile-per-hour winds, and possibly more than a foot of snow in some areas. This would be the first day we would encounter any sort of mountain driving. We approached the Black Hills. I remembered this area from when I was kid. I had been fascinated with Deadwood where all the old famous cowboy's graves were. It was now a major tourist area with casinos. I wished we could stop and explore the town, but we were getting more and more aggressive about pushing on.

The Black Hills were easy to maneuver. Going up in elevation was not scary at all because the fastest the truck would go was about 35 miles per hour up steep grades. Tommy was sleeping as we reached a point that seemed like it was at the edge of the planet. There were no towns, no truck stops, and the landscape was barren aside from some sage brush. There was some snow up there, but the roads were clear. Tommy woke up about the same time I started to panic about running out of gas. We pulled into a truck stop just as the gas light went on. I did most of the driving again that day—a fact I'm very proud of. We switched drivers in Buffalo, Wyoming, at the foot of the Big Horn mountains. We got gas, lunch, and used the facilities all at the same time. We were getting more efficient at this. I think it was here Tommy revealed the obvious fact that he was more nervous when I was driving then when he was. I didn't care. I felt like I was becoming a pro by then.

We did not drive into the Big Horn Mountains. The interstate actually goes around them. That was probably good because that was where all the snow had fallen the night before. Buffalo had a little bit of snow, but most of it had already melted. This marked the halfway point of our trip. We were really enjoying it now.

We found our motel in Billings just as it was getting dark. The weather was warmer but very drizzly. This Super 8 had the pet fee, but we were able to leave the room. We returned to the room after another Happy Chef meal. We called family to let them know we had made it that far safely. It was refreshing to hear familiar voices other than our own. We were planning a big drive the next day. If things went well, we would try to get to Spokane, Washington. We were headed for the Rocky Mountains, though, and it was tough to tell what weather we would encounter.

DAY FOUR

This time when we left the room, we left one of the dresser drawers open. When we returned Mosely was hiding inside the dresser drawer. We had the cats figured out as well as they had figured out our routine. On to Spokane!

I knew I was destined to do at least some of the mountain driving. I studied the map the night before and realized I might even have to go over the Continental Divide. Once we started, it was clear that weather was not going to be a problem. That was a relief! I also realized that driving in the mountains was not going to be a problem for me. The worst part was going downhill. Traveling at a 6% grade looking straight downhill with 11,000 pounds behind you and on wheels gave the word "freefall" a whole new meaning. Tommy thought I was a little bit heavy on the brakes. There was a real danger to that, too. Apparently, the brakes can become hot and completely useless. That fact was not comforting. Other than that, the day was uneventful to this point. We both enjoyed the driving and the wonderful scenery. If we weren't so excited about Seattle, we'd actually have extended this trip.

We arrived in Missoula, Montana, our original destination, at about 2:00 p.m. We were really cruising now. Meals had become somewhat less important. We stopped at a truck stop for gas and had frozen burritos for lunch. I was somewhat nauseated by the taste and some of the mysterious ingredients. But once again, this trip was not for wimps. We had to push on! We cancelled the reservation in Missoula and made a new one in Spokane.

Some of the most challenging mountain passes were in Idaho of all places. Fortunately, Tommy was driving at this point, although, I must admit it was also nerve-wracking sitting in the passenger seat since he was much more conservative with the brakes. Again, the freefall experience. Those passes even had ramps to stop runaway trucks. That was comforting! The drive was beautiful, though.

We arrived in Spokane at a reasonable time and found the motel without a hitch. This Super 8 did not have a Happy Chef, so we were forced to venture out for dinner. We had reached a city with ethnic restaurants! The Seattle influence could be seen at this stage of our journey. We pulled into an auto parts store's parking lot to turn around, and there was an espresso cart in the middle of the lot! Our meal, with wine, at the Italian restaurant we chose for dinner was a bit pricey, but we thought we definitely deserved it, especially since we had those frozen burritos for lunch. We discussed how excited we were about the last day of our journey. Could we really be this close?

DAY FIVE

We got a wake-up call at 6:00 a.m. We ate breakfast at a nearby restaurant and were on the road by 8:00 a.m. We hoped to get to Seattle by around noon. The drive through western Washington was mostly desert. Missile sites and the radioactive Hanford Site were located here. An ominous thought. This looked nothing like the part of Washington where we would live. It was almost noon before we hit the Cascade Range, which eventually dropped down to Seattle. Just a couple more mountain passes, and we would be there. There was snow in the mountains. We passed Roslyn, Washington, where the show "Northern Exposure" was filmed. It looked like northern Wisconsin, only much bigger. We stopped in a small town to call our apartment building, use the restroom, and visit a small espresso shop. We were really close to Seattle now! At about 2:00 p.m., we reached the outlying suburbs of Seattle. It did not look like your standard suburbia. Homes hugged the western slopes of the Cascade Range, and fir trees were still very thick at this point. It was a very subtle approach into Seattle. It began to look more like suburbia as we got into Bellevue. We crossed Lake Washington and Mercer Island and entered a tunnel with much anticipation. Buju Banton's dancehall reggae was blaring on the stereo. (We had now listened to every single tape in our collection.) There was light at the end of the tunnel. We were out of the tunnel! We were there! We could now see the Seattle skyline. In fact, we were rapidly approaching the center of the city. We now had to focus on the exact location of our apartment and how to get there. We decided the best thing to do was to drive downtown and connect with the numbered streets until we found 2nd Street where we would live. Tommy did a great job of driving the truck through downtown traffic. The next big hurdle was parking. There really wasn't a great place to park a big truck with a car in the middle of the city—and how were we going to unload everything? Fortunately, there were three unoccupied parking spots about one block from our apartment building.

It was now three o'clock and we had a truck to unload that had to be back sometime the same evening. I didn't even know how we were going to unload it given the fact that we were parked one block away. I decided to call the truck company to get exact directions and find out how late we could return it. To our relief, we had until midnight to drop the keys off. This still seemed like an impossible task. I was very stressed, and I could tell Tommy was, too, but we just had to get through this one last challenge. We were told we could pull the truck into the narrow alley behind the building and unload our goods into the parking garage. I don't know what seemed more precarious—the narrowness of the alley and the potential of having to move the truck should someone need to get through, or the street people in the alley eyeing us up along with all our possessions. There was nothing to do but start unloading. Worrying at this point was not going to solve anything.

The back end of the truck was loaded with all the last stuff to go in—all the loose odds and ends, cleaning supplies, etc. You never realize how much junk you have until you load it into a truck like that. After about two hours, the truck was completely unloaded. We were physically and mentally exhausted, since we did not eat lunch or breakfast that day. The adrenaline was pumping and was the only thing keeping us going. We didn't see how it would be physically possible for us to get our stuff up the elevator and to our apartment given our state. We worried about this for just a minute and then dug right in again. We devised a plan where I would move everything to the elevator and Tommy would take it up and to the room. This was working quite well, and after about an hour, we began to see some headway. I can remember moments when I felt I was actually going to faint. I wasn't being a wimp—Tommy said the same thing! I don't think I've ever done that level of activity for such a long time. It was around 10:30 p.m. when we got all the boxes into our apartment. Although everything was still in boxes,

we made sure to set up our bed properly because we would be sleeping-in the next morning. We still had to take the truck back to a strange suburb, which seemed a million miles away. We spent a few minutes collecting our thoughts and orienting ourselves on the map in our very disoriented state. I was afraid that we were in no condition to take the truck back. But there was just this last thing, and then we were done.

Finding the truck company wasn't that difficult. There was a very helpful man there who helped us fill out our paperwork and unhook our car. After Tommy went through what seemed like an endless mass of paperwork, we were ready to go. I was glad he was still functioning enough to handle that part because I was falling asleep in the chair. It was such a relief to be driving our car without the truck. I felt like our feet were finally on the ground. We arrived at our apartment, drank some wine to celebrate (this seemed like a necessary ritual, although we were almost too tired to do even that). The cats seemed happy. They seemed to know this stop was different. There would be no long drive tomorrow. Now for the endless sleep....

I think it was about a week before we felt like ourselves again. The disoriented state probably lasted another two or three days. Our legs were peppered with bruises, which took four or five days to go away. It took one week before we had everything unpacked. Amazingly nothing got broken. There are a couple of small things that we haven't found yet. It was at this point when we started the next big adventure—exploring the new city.

CHAPTER 2
A Flicker of a Heartbeat

Carole

It wasn't until three years later I received the news from Stacey that I was going to be a grandmother, and that is when I began to save her e-mails.

Subject: Hello from Seattle
Date: Fri, 19 Jun 1998

Hi, Mom and Gary,

Just wanted to drop you a quick line and let you know that my ultrasound appointment went fine today.

It's too early for them to say that "I am in the clear," but everything looked great. I got to see a flicker of a heartbeat. Am very proud to be carrying his/her first baby picture (really just a blur on the screen!). Other than that, I am super tired and a little queasy in the mornings until 10:30 or so. I can usually handle some cinnamon toast and a little juice but that's it.

It's supposed to be a nice weekend here. Maybe I'll muster up enough energy for a hike. Maybe not. Look forward to talking to you.

Love, Stacey

Subject: Goodbye summer in Seattle
Date: Wed, 30 Sep 1998

Hi, Mom and Gary,

I'm off work a little early today, so I get to enjoy the last bits of daylight.

Actually, I was going to go back to work after my doctor's appointment, but I got on the wrong bus and ended up on the freeway. I couldn't get off until Boeing Field. At least that ended my moral dilemma (whether I should go back in or play hooky).

My appointment went fine. My doctor was in her normal rush, but I did manage to sit her down long enough to answer my questions. We listened to the heartbeat again. Everything was good and normal. I've gained an incredible 10 lbs. over the last six weeks. It seems like a lot to me, but the nurse said it was about right. I made sure they did a blood test this time, I don't trust this managed care. I think sometimes they try to skimp on these tests.

I narrowed down options for flights in November. I'm still sad we can't stay longer, I'm really homesick, and these pregnancy hormones don't help!

Love, Stacey

Subject: Re: Hi from Mom
Date: Tue, 13 Oct 1998

Hi, Mom and Gary,

Tommy and I just got home from a hospital birthing suite tour and a pizza dinner. It's 8:00, and I'm pretty exhausted. The hospital rooms were nicer than I expected. They have 17 suites. I've heard they can run out if you are unlucky. There were fabulous views of the Sound in the room we looked at. There is also a Jacuzzi in the private bathroom in each room. We got to see a tiny newborn in the nursery.

Love, Stacey

By the winter of 1998, Stacey had changed jobs and was working for the Environmental Home Center in Seattle, a company that promotes "green living" and provides eco-friendly solutions for homes and businesses.

Subject: Re: It's cooollddd here! Ditto.
Date: Tue, 22 Dec 1998

Hi, Mom and Gary,

Got your e-mail. I was feeling sorry for myself because it was so cold today. I forget what -30 and -50 feels like. It was 17 this morning, not quite as bad as you have it, but very unusual for Seattle.

My workplace was 59 degrees this morning. I think at times it warmed to 64. The water in the toilet was frozen, and yesterday our pipes were frozen. My boss is pretty understanding. He let everyone leave an hour early today. I came home and took a warm bath. It was the first time I was warm all day. We are supposed to have a chance for a considerable amount of snow on Christmas Eve. I'm a little worried because we are leaving for Portland. We'll try to play it smart, perhaps leaving a little earlier or later than expected. The worst thing that could happen is we don't go, and we have to forfeit our reservations for the first night.

I will call on Christmas, hopefully from Portland! Have a nice Christmas Eve. Wish we could be there.

Love, Stacey

Subject: Re: Grandma flies to Seattle, Yipppeeeeeee!
Date: Tue, 29 Dec 1998

Hi, Mom,

I got your e-mail. I'm sorry you ended up paying more for your ticket. It sounds like you got the times you wanted, though. I don' t think you will have to spend much money once you're here. We can get you to the airport and back easily, we'll cover for the guest suite, and we should have a full stock of food in the cupboards. It will be so nice to share this wonderful time with you!

I have had terrible insurance problems. I found out last week that my doctor is not on my company's new plan (even though she is listed in their book). I've been fighting the insurance company ever since. I thought everything was straightened out yesterday and was quite shocked when my doctor's office at first refused to see me today. After a few more calls to the insurance company and a few embarrassing tears in the reception area, they let me in! It's awful that you have to fight for your right to see your doctor. Managed care really stinks!

I hope that you have a good New Year's. We have no plans yet. We will probably go out for an anniversary dinner. If I take a nap, I will be able to stay up and watch the fireworks. They shoot them off the top of the Space Needle. We've never been around to see this, but I guess the view is great from our roof.

Love, Stacey

Subject: names??????
Date: Wed, 6 Jan 1999

Hi, Mom and Gary,

Tommy told me I was supposed to run this name by the grandparents. What do you think of Alexander Thomas Lesiewicz (Alex Lesiewicz)???

Hope you're having fun in the winter wonderland. Everything is fine out here, still growing. I had another pregnant picture to send you, but Tommy accidentally deleted it. I'm thinking it may not have been an accident. He says he'll take another one. I'll talk to you soon.

Love, Stacey

Subject: Baby report
Date: Tue, 19 Jan. 1999

Hi, Mom and Gary,

Had my doctor's appointment today. Everything seems good. She said I am the picture-perfect size. This was good to hear because

I am tired of people saying I look small. No dilation, but I'm 50% effaced so the contractions have been doing some work. She also recommended that we pack our hospital bags and put the car seat in the car, just in case....

I got a little freaked this weekend about everything that we need to do. I got a lot of work done on the baby's room, so I think I feel better.

Can't wait to see you. I think that the next month will be a whirlwind, so it won't seem like long.

Love, Stacey

Subject: Baby report
Date: Tue, 9 Feb 1999

Hello, Everyone,

I had my weekly appointment this afternoon. Baby is healthy and happy. My doctor estimates that his size will be around 8 lbs. I had no idea I was expecting a big baby, I guess that is still in the average range. She is talking about induction on the 20th if I don't have the baby before then. I'm not thrilled about the thought of that but hopefully things will go naturally. She said to walk a lot. I'll have to hike down to the market tomorrow in our brisk 35-degree weather—brrrrrrrrrrrr.

I finished packing for the hospital. I have so much stuff, it's a little embarrassing. We will need to pull up to the emergency exit in a U-Haul if I bring anything else. The funniest thing I have is this big rubber exercise ball. I went to the gas station to fill it with air. (I put gas in the car, too.) Everyone says they are great to bounce around on when you're in labor. Can you imagine?

I went down to my garden this afternoon. The chard looks beautiful, and I have daffodils and tulips coming up. It may be a while before I get back down there.

Love, Stacey

Aleks Thomas Lesiewicz was born February 13, 1999.

Subject: Re: Smiles
Date: Tue, 9 Mar 1999

He smiled at me! First last night when he was in the swing. He just started waking up, and I thought I would go to him before he fussed, and out came this cute little smile.

Today after fussing in the swing, I went on the "bouncy ball" with him, and I got three really genuine smiles as he looked at me. It was so cute. This is really going to be fun!

Love, Stacey

Subject: Hello from Stacey
Date: Wed, 21 Apr 1999

I think your grandson is going to be a "cut-up" just like his dad. We went to our PEPS group today (new parent support group), and he tried to be the center of attention any way he could. First, he farted very loudly three times while other women were telling their birth stories. He turned some heads each time! Then we had to sing a little song. It went like this "Hello, (baby's name). How do you do? Stay right there, and we'll clap for you!" When they got to Aleks, he made a great big smile. Most of the babies were oblivious.

I'm excited about this group. It seems like a great bunch of women. We will meet weekly in each other's homes. Finally, a way to make friends in this city! I also plan to begin postnatal yoga in May. We bring our babies to class. I'm not sure how much yoga will be accomplished, but I could sure use it.

Matt put me on the back burner for work again. He postponed our meeting to next Thursday. He says that things have just been chaos around there. Don't miss it at all!

I am very disturbed about what happened in Denver as I'm sure all of you teachers are. We have a friend that teaches in a Denver suburb. It's just insane. Well, Aleks is awake. Time to go.

Love, Stacey

Subject: Re: Hello from Grandma
Date: Sat, 24 Apr 1999

Aleks and I did get out for a nature hike yesterday. We had to drive to Discovery Park, and then I took him in the sling. Anyway, he woke up from a nap and he was under all of these trees. His eyes opened wide with amazement. I think he thought the world was all concrete and linear shapes. I guess that was my Earth Day thing introducing him to nature. It's been awhile since I've sat under a tree, too.

Love, Stacey

Subject: Re: Hi from Mom
Date: Fri, 13 Aug 1999

Hi,

I think he is more or less crawling. I took a video of it yesterday, and Tom and I would both classify it as a first crawl. The cats have a jittery look of panic. Yesterday Aleks came bounding across the floor head on with Creepy. He had this silly smile on his face and was looking right in Creepy's eyes. Creepy started to take defensive action just as I intercepted. I don't look forward to the day they have a confrontation.

I got some childproofing devices now that I know anything in the room below 18 inches is a target. Today it was the phone books. We lost the last two pages of our Z's. Oh, well.

Time to go. Someone is sucking on my ankle and wants my attention.

Love, Stacey

Subject: Re: Happy Tuesday
Date: Wed, 18 Aug 1999

Hi, Mom,

Aleks continues to refine his crawling skills. His favorite toys now are speaker wire, stroller wheels, anything paper, the cat food dishes, remote controls, the battery charger, and shoes. He gets so pissed off because I won't let him have any of these things. He likes it when Daddy comes home. Daddy is a lot more fun and easy-going. Daddy let him get too close to Creepy yesterday. You can guess what happened. Fortunately, it wasn't too serious of a confrontation. I think the only one who learned a lesson was Daddy.

Love, Stacey

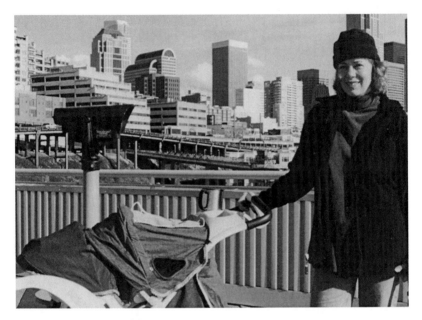

Date: Wed, 8 Sep 1999

Aleks woke up early, wide awake at 5:00 a.m. Went back to sleep at 7:15 after Tom left and slept until 10:15. Boy, did that feel good! We went to the market today and bought tons of produce. Now I have to cook! Enjoyed some violin players at the market—they did some Mozart pieces. Aleks is now in his "dropping" stage. It's not a good idea to give him my wallet as a teether. Found this out today. Fortunately, I still have my wallet and credit cards!

I'm talking to my boss tomorrow. Tommy and I talked last night. After some thought, I really want to limit my working. It's stressing us both out. Can't do it at night anymore. We both need time to relax. I hope he [boss] understands. I can continue to do 10 hours a week, but we're thinking I may even need help with that. I may see if one of two women in the building will do two hours a day, four hours a week so that I can work, or exercise, or get my hair cut, or go to the dentist.

Love, Stacey

Subject: Re: Hello from Mom
Date: Wed, 22 Sep 1999

Hi, Mom,

The baby sitting went really well today after a tough day yesterday. I have been getting caught up on my work. Two hours seems just right. The weather has been so nice that I've been taking my work up to the deck and working out there. What a luxury!

As far as new things for Aleks…. I have been giving him puffed rice cereal for fun. He mostly plays with those and leaves a trail everywhere. Tommy fed him some banana slices on Sunday not knowing they should be chopped small. I came home (luckily) and saw Aleks eating them. He had his mouth loaded up like 737's waiting for take-off on the runway at O'Hare. I took one slice out, and another popped out and another. I have to give Tommy credit, though. He is a good dad.

I plan to take a picture of him standing for you, He is pulling up on everything.

Love, Stacey

CHAPTER 3

Lesley and Jon Join the Peace Corps

On October 4, 1999, a daughter, Kyli, was born in New Orleans to Stacey's stepbrother, Cary and his wife, Jill.

Stacey's sister Lesley and husband Jon left the States in September of that year for Africa to begin training as Peace Corps volunteers.

Subject: Hi from Seattle
Date: Wed, 6 Oct 1999

Any more details about our new little Southern belle? When do you go to New Orleans? Is it this weekend or next? I'll bet you're anxious.

Loved the letter from Lesley. Thanks for forwarding it. It sounds like she is surrounded by nice, loving people not to mention a fabulous setting. Made me teary-eyed....

Aleks discovered the volume control on the stereo this week and the button to turn the vacuum on and off. Both scare him, but I was able to demonstrate cause and effect to him. He thinks it's funny when I turn the stereo volume up but cries when it happens to him.

I called his pediatrician about his night waking yesterday. She says it is separation anxiety. Says they suggest reading the Ferber (cry it out book.) She didn't try anything like that on her own kids until after one year. She had a few gentler suggestions as well. Tom got up with him a couple of times on Sunday night. It's nice to have that support. I know it's hard for him to do on work nights. We have a very rigid bedtime routine, which now involves a little bath and some nice warm jammies. He was in bed at 7:30 and slept until 2:30. I nursed him, and he was back to sleep in 15 minutes. That was the only time he woke up. We put one of my shirts in bed with him, I also did not turn on the heat and the blinds were up, so it was lighter in the room. Oh, and his friends, My Buddy, Maximillian, Pooh, and Little Kitty, were all watching over him. All things we will try again tonight....

Love, Stacey

Letter from Lesley
Wednesday, September 22, 1999
Lesley Reynolds, PCT
Corps de la Paix
Lomé, Togo
Afrique de l'Ouest

Hello, Everybody,

A lot has happened over the last four or five days, so it will be hard for me to remember all of the experiences I have been having. Training has been very time-consuming so far, and it's not very easy for me to find time to write letters or write in my journal.

Unfortunately, Jon and I had to split up into our training groups on Sunday the 19th. He, for the next 11 weeks, is in a town called Kuma Dunyo, and I am in Agou. We still are going to be able to be together on Thursdays, Saturdays and Sundays.

The ride to my village was about 1-1/2 hours long, and there was a lot to see on the way. We went through a lot of checkpoints, but the gendarmes must automatically let the Peace Corps vans through because we didn't have to stop. The area of Togo that my village is in is absolutely beautiful. Almost like paradise. It's very mountainous and extremely lush There are mango trees, banana trees, papaya trees, and flowers everywhere.

When my group arrived in the village of Agou-Agbetsiko, the welcome was incredible. A band with horns and drums started a procession that led us into the village. I think the entire town was surrounding us. Everyone was singing and dancing to the music. The singing was in Ewe, so I'm not sure what the singing was about. Eventually the procession ended at the entrance to the village. At this point, some of the village elders dressed in traditional Togolese robes stopped and faced everyone. One of the men began to pray. While he was praying, he poured water on the ground three times—once for a blessing for us, once for the people of the village, and once for the ancestors. Although he was praying in Ewe, one of the Togolese men who works for the Peace Corps explained that he was blessing our arrival in his prayers and praying that our efforts in Togo will be successful.

After the prayers, the music and singing started up again, and we danced into a shelter. Inside the shelter, our luggage was all piled up in a circle in the middle. The dancing continued, and soon I realized we were dancing around our luggage. Pretty strange! It was definitely a lot of fun, though.

At the end of the ceremony, we were matched up with our host family for training. I was matched up with Alomadou Tsalevo and his wife, Madame Alomadou. He is 59 years old, and she is 57. They have three children. The oldest is 35 and the youngest is 19. None of the children live at home anymore, but there are two kids who live with them, a girl who is seven and a boy who is five. I think the children are a niece and nephew, but I haven't quite figured it out. So far, the family has been extremely generous and very patient with my less-than-perfect French skills. They built me my very own outhouse in the backyard the first day I was here, and they spent an hour putting up the mosquito net in my room and making sure it was just right. I have my own room with a bed and a table. The Peace Corps is bringing in either a bigger bed or another smaller bed this week so Jon can stay here. I don't have electricity or running water (some of the other trainees in my village have both!), so I use a lantern for light and take bucket showers outside. The bucket showers are great, though, especially in the morning when the sun is coming up and I'm surrounded by huge palm trees and banana trees... Ahhh!!! It's really nice. There is music in the distance, too. Not radio music but real, live music. It's usually horns or drums, and sometimes there is singing also.

The food has been pretty good so far. They trained the host families about boiling our water and preparing food using good hygiene but compared to American standards (and what our feeble little American bodies are used to), I think the basic food handling and food preparation are not very safe. I have been making the mistake of watching Madame Alomadou make dinner in her little dirt floor kitchen. It's pretty scary, but I haven't gotten sick yet. I had fufu for the first time tonight. It's pretty good. Other than that, I have been eating a lot of rice and beans, corn paté with tomato sauce, bread, and fruit.

In the morning, I leave for Peace Corps training at seven. It's about a twenty-minute walk to the training center, so I usually walk with another Peace Corps person. There are a lot of market stands set up along the way. It's fun to look at all of the things for sale. Today I bought some flip-flops on the way to class. We are in class until 5:45 p.m., which makes for a really long day. Lately we have been stopping at a bar called Afrikoko on the way home from class (usually four or five Peace Corp people). It's a funky, brightly colored "buvette" with outdoor seating and really good reggae music. Every time we stop, I get an orange soda (in a bottle), but they do have quite a few different kinds of beer (even Guinness!! I can't wait to take Jon there).

It is still the rainy season here. The day our group arrived in the village was the first day it hadn't rained in months. The people in the village said it was a "good sign." It doesn't rain all day, though. Usually there will be two really heavy downpours a day and the rest of the day will be sunny and hot. It is super humid here already, and I guess this is the cool season.

There are animals all over the place in my village. It's kind of annoying at times—goats, chickens, cats and dogs everywhere. I get the impression they just belong to whoever wants them.

The two little kids that live in my house are absolutely in love with me. They come into my room every night and watch me read and sometimes they sit next to me and pet my hair! It's pretty cute!

Well, I guess I better go now—I have to study a little French. Tomorrow is Thursday so I get to see Jon! :) I can't wait.

Take care and send a package soon! Hints for package: M&M's, liquid hand sanitizer, hard candy, power bars, pictures of family and our wedding.

Love you lots!! Lesley

To: All
Lesley and Jon News #6 10-25-99

For those of you who have not yet heard the news, we are back in the United States. For some people, it was not a big shock to hear we were back, and for some, it was quite a surprise.

We just want everyone to know that we don't regret going to Togo at all. It was a wonderful experience for us, and we learned a lot. Overall, there wasn't one main reason that we came home.... a lot of little things contributed to our decision to return. Basically, there were more things pulling us back here than keeping us there. And our health was a little bit compromised. (Lesley found out she has a parasite—a little piece of Togo that will stay with her for a while!!!)

For now, we are heading back to Chicago. We have an apartment lined up to move into on Nov. 15. Lesley is going back to her job at the hospital, and Jon is currently applying/ interviewing for a new job (the commute to Barrington was something he didn't want to come back to). We are excited to be going back to Chicago.... it kinda feels like where we belong right now. Sometimes you have to get really far away from where you are (8,000 miles) to put everything into perspective and realize that is the place where you belong. Take care, everyone.

Jon and Lesley

CHAPTER 4
SWAT Teams and Tear Gas

Subject: mama
Date: Fri, 8 Oct 1999

Hi,

Hope you had a nice week. We had Seattle weather here in true form. Misty rain. I think Aleks will have to get used to the rain. To be true Seattleites, we will need to go out regardless. Only on the blusteriest days will we stay in and try to amuse ourselves.

We visited a daycare center today. I thought I'd go see the one that came most recommended by people I know. They have an infant opening. I didn't run away screaming, but I came to the conclusion that it would not be the best environment for Aleks now.... That makes my decision-making easier in that I have eliminated one option. It looks like it is home care of some type or I don't work. My boss is willing to make my position a little more focused and lucrative by having me work less at a higher hourly rate. I will forfeit the opportunity to make commissions (big bucks if it ever happens). I'm also getting more help from the rest of the staff. We'll see....

Next weekend is our little family trip to the coast. We will have four days and will travel just north of Victoria, BC. It should be fun.

I think he is officially saying mama. If I leave the room, he crawls after me muttering, "Mama, mama," and it is typical to hear it if he is crying in his crib, making him totally irresistible. I just have to pick him up. Love that little guy.

Stacey (mama)

Subject: trip
Date: Tue, 19 Oct 1999

Hi,

We are back in the states after Aleks' first out-of-country experience. We decided to take the later ferry back from Victoria. We got home at about 8:30 last night.

What a splendid weekend. The leaves were peaking. It was warm, in the 60's. No winds. The Strait of Juan de Fuca looked like glass most of the time. We were really lucky.

We had to rush to catch the ferry Friday morning. Aleks' cold seemed a little better, but I made sure to pack all the gear (vaporizer, Tylenol, nasal aspirator). We stayed in Victoria Friday night and the next morning walked around the city and found a really good health food restaurant. Aleks is so easy to travel with at the present time. He sleeps in the car and is good in restaurants as long as you give him some Cheerios or something else to chew on. Everyone in Victoria seemed to love him in spite of his snotty nose.

We travelled west of Victoria one hour to Point No Point. We arrived at 4:00 check-in time. Our unit was a shared duplex unit (I thought we had an individual unit). We expressed a little concern because of the baby waking up at night. They assured us it was sound-proof and not to worry. This is a place where people, mostly couples, go to get away from it all. No TVs, no phones. I thought the units or little cabins were designed really well. They overlooked the strait with open ocean out beyond. Waves crashed on a rocky beach below us. The view could be enjoyed from the deck with hot tub, through a large picture window in the living room in front of a small wood burning fireplace, or from the sleeping loft upstairs. The sun set over the Olympic Mountains to our southwest exactly in the middle of our picture window.

The first night, Aleks went to sleep early, so Tommy and I plugged in the baby monitor and hit the hot tub with some champagne. It was a gorgeous night to look up at the stars from the tub. We went to bed pretty early, about 10:30 or so. I fell asleep reflecting on how easy it was to travel with a baby. Things had not changed too much. Then Aleks woke up at 11:30, 12:30, 1:00, and between 2 and 4. In fact, he did not sleep much at all that night. His congestion wasn't bad, and he didn't seem sick. He just wanted to eat. We were worried about his crying, so, of course, we had to yield to his every whimper. I think I slept three hours that night. I felt like heck the next day, but of course, it was too nice a day to waste napping, so I muscled my way through it. It was a beautiful day—the weather, showing Aleks cool new things.

On Sunday night, Aleks still did not sleep well. Not as bad as the night before, and we were able to sleep in Monday morning since we decided not to try for the early ferry.

We spent some more time in Victoria before hitting the 4:00 ferry. In fact, we were having so much fun buying Aleks toys and silly hats we almost forgot about the ferry.

Love, Stacey

Subject: happy midweek
Date: Wed, 10 Nov 1999

Hello,

We had our baby class today. It was a fun thing to do on a very rainy day. Two veteran mothers of four in the class asked me if I realize I'm going to have a walker very soon.

After class, Aleks and I went to Sears to buy a "big boy" car seat, and then I stopped in at work. I have three big projects coming to a head now. I think I can handle them if that is all I focus on other than my obvious responsibilities.

Tommy and Aleks went to the homeowners meeting tonight. I guess they are preparing the building for the WTO conference in a couple of weeks. They have to lock up the decks fearing that protestors may hang banners or propel themselves off the top. Already there have been suspicious people asking for access. It should be an exciting time around here. The labor halls are all in our neighborhood. The union halls are planning a huge march during two days of the conference. They told us to treat those days as a snow emergency—don't plan to drive around and perhaps stock up on essentials. The main conference, which will have world leaders from everywhere, maybe even Fidel Castro, is not too close to our place. It is right by Tommy's work. Most of that part of town will be shut down for four or five days. Aleks and I will probably keep a low profile, so you won't have to worry.

Subject: Hello from Seattle
Date: Fri, 19 Nov 1999

Hello,

Tommy and I had a fun night out. We went to see B.B. King at the Paramount Theatre. We stopped for a microbrew and appetizers on the way and ran into one of our friends, Rob Harrison. He is the architect who does sustainable design, and he goes for motorcycle rides with Tommy. So, we both have a lot in common with him.

The concert was great. I'm glad we saw B.B. He's been playing for 50 years. I doubt he will be playing too much longer.

Aleks did fine with the sitter. She said that she thought he was sad about our absence. He crawled into our bedroom and looked around with sort of a bewildered look. She said he was real serious but didn't cry much. She put him to sleep in kind of an unorthodox way. She took him on the roof and rocked him in the stroller.

Love, Stacey

Subject: Re: WTO
Date: Sun, 28 Nov 1999

We had a nice sunny day here in Seattle even though at 2:00 the sun was so low in the sky you could not even feel it. The days are getting pretty short here at the 48th latitude. After yoga, I took

Aleks out for a long walk in the stroller. We went downtown and to the market to see what kind of excitement was brewing. There were some protestors in front of The Gap and some planes with banners. Lots of police on the street. Not too many people out today, though. I think many would-be shoppers stayed home.

We will stay close to home and not go out in the car for the next three days because traffic will be crazy. Tuesday is the big demonstration. It will go down 4th Avenue between the Space Needle and Convention Center, just two blocks from our house. Aleks and I will probably watch it from the roof. We should have a good view, and we will be safe from that vantage point. I would consider going to the march if my sitter came that day, but she has decided not to brave the traffic and will come later. Tommy and I will probably go out for a little dinner.

Tommy will really be in the thick of things. His building is practically connected to the Convention Center where the WTO is being held. He thinks that everyone is making too big of a deal of it.

Love, Stacey

Date: Mon, 29 Nov 1999

Tom is going to work tomorrow. He said only ten were in his office today. The most interesting demonstration will be in the morning when they chain themselves together to try to keep the conference from starting. He will probably see that on his way in. I'm sure that protestors will be gathering when Aleks and I go for coffee at my favorite spot by the Space Needle. We will be safe on our doorstep by the time the huge march takes place. I guess they will not allow us on the roof due to security. We will have to watch from ground level, if at all.

Love, Stacey

Subject: wow, this is weird
Date: Tue, 30 Nov 1999

Hi, folks in Boscobel.

The streets of Seattle are pretty strange right now. Aleks and I went to get coffee this morning but didn't go too far. I've been watching continuous coverage on TV and calling to inform Tommy when they were tear-gassing outside of his building.

Stacey

Subject: tear gassed in Seattle
Date: Tue, 30 Nov 1999

Tommy and I went out for dinner tonight since our sitter decided to come tonight instead of during the day. I insisted on a drink at the Cyclops (across the street), and then we were to go to a restaurant by the market. We left the Cyclops and headed for the market. Suddenly and mysteriously, we both started to sneeze. Then we noticed that other pedestrians coming from that direction were covering their noses. Then it hit us. Apparently, it was tear gas wafting in the air. It really stung!

We are fine and safe here in spite of what it looks like on the media. Tommy is working in Bellevue tomorrow. Aleks and I probably will not go to our class. They are protesting at the university we go to.

Love, Stacey

Subject: Hello from Seattle
Date: Wed, 1 Dec 1999

Hi, everyone,

Just wanted to let you know we survived the wild day yesterday. Things were actually quiet around our building throughout the day and night even though much of the action was only blocks away.

Tommy was in the thick of it at work. Some of the most volatile demonstrations were outside of his building. As usual, he played it down. He said the protesters actually helped him through the crowds.

The Labor March was beautiful with people of all ages and every cause you can imagine taking part. It is too bad that later others chose to take advantage of the situation.

Today promises to be different, it sounds like the police and National Guard will take a strong-arm approach so things should not deteriorate like they did yesterday.

Aleks and I will stick close to home and watch the events, if any, unfold on TV.

Love you all, Stacey

Subject: Seattle, a view from the inside
Date: Thu, 2 Dec 1999

Hello,

I finally decided to venture out with Aleks today. We were really getting cabin fever after literally being shut in for two days. The sun was out, and the wind had died down from this morning. We walked briskly towards the downtown core "curfew zone." As I got closer, a feeling of relief swept over me because things seemed really normal. The streets were full of shoppers and business people. The only thing really unusual was the large contingent of police in the Westlake Center mall. The entire mall was filled with police cars, and police in riot gear surrounded the area. From what I had seen on the news, the latest protesters were gathering on Capitol Hill about a mile away. It was an eerie feeling pushing a baby stroller in front of those police, but they were actually nice and were laughing at Aleks' funny hat. Perhaps the strangest thing about downtown was the boarded-up shops—Nike Town, Pottery Barn, Gap, Nordstrom, everything. No more Christmas trains or Santas for Aleks and me to look at in the windows!

Hunger pangs began to lead me to the market to get one of my favorite burritos. I looked for an ATM to get some cash. The first one I went to was not working—it had been damaged in the riot. I crossed Westlake again in front of the police and found the next one in working order. With cash in my pocket, we headed towards the market. I was also looking forward to getting a little Christmas shopping done. I haven't even started it. I popped into a small store and started looking at some earrings. A timid shopkeeper approached me and said the police had just been through to warn the shops of an impending demonstration. The Pike Street Market had just been closed down again. We talked a little more about the last couple of days, and both agreed that more than anything we were afraid of the tear gas that has been used in tremendous amounts. It's the last thing I would want Aleks messed up in. I was close to a purchasing decision but could not make up my mind because, (a) I was really hungry, (b) I could feel myself beginning to sweat, and (c) I was becoming very distracted by the police sirens outside and the motorcycle brigade that had just gone by. Time to get my little boy home. I was outta there!

As I walked down First Avenue towards home, I could look down to the market in one direction and see the swell of people gathering and chanting. I could see police loaded up in all types of vehicles. I picked up the pace. Once I felt we were in the "safe zone," I checked out another burrito place. It was closed. Was it due to the demonstrations? Were the owners out protesting? Who knows?

Down the street closer to home, I swung into the bakery and got a sandwich. Aleks was sleeping. Even if I didn't get any shopping done, I had accomplished that!

At home I turned on the TV to see what was going on down the street. I was a victim of paranoia. I found out the demonstration in the market was large but very peaceful. It was all about family farms. The march will head this direction later. They will have a police escort instead of mass arrests.

I thought maybe I would support some small local shops and artisans this Christmas in the spirit of the anti-WTO stance, but actually online shopping is beginning to look more and more attractive....

For this afternoon, I think Aleks and I will focus on something else. We're just sick of this. Maybe we will go for a swim.

Love, Stacey

CHAPTER 5
Doc Martens and Earrings

Subject: Re: Hi from Mom
Date: Sat, 22 Jan 2000

Our nanny is coming for the last time on Tuesday. I decided to keep looking for other avenues. She was getting along with Aleks well, but I still was a little uncomfortable. One day I came home to a very dirty diaper with no evidence of being changed in the 4.5-5 hours I was gone. I was wimpy and just told her our job situations were changing.

They are looking for another designer at work. I guess they are placing ads. Hopefully I will have help there soon. I would like to work as little as possible for a while. For a sitter, I may advertise at the Art Institute and Antioch University. Perhaps a student would be interested in coming a couple of hours a day. I'm also going to see if the cleaning lady can come to clean once a week. I'm doing some deep cleaning now because as it stands, I would be too embarrassed to have someone do it. I have been a "clutter buster" this weekend.

Tommy had time off on Thursday and Friday between jobs. He has been spending a lot of time with AleklllZ'q"l'l'l' ll'1lll"'al (Aleks is helping!) He starts his new job on Monday. I think he is excited.

We went car shopping yesterday. I think we are going to get a wagon. A real family car!! Today we decided we must wait a couple of weeks. Our lives are too crazy to worry about doing a test drive and lining up financing.

The washing machine repair guy just left. Seems our washer is shot. We will need to replace it ASAP. All of our appliances seem to be on the blink, including our dishwasher and TV. Having a washer and dishwasher that don't work is hard on me, but when the TV doesn't work, I get more work out of Tommy! I guess it balances. Don't tell him I said that.

Love, Stacey

Subject: Greetings from Seattle
Date: Thu, 27 Jan 2000

Tommy loves his new job. I really think he is making it all up and doesn't have a job. It sounds too good to be true. I hope things go well. It sounds very relaxed. On his first day, they watched one of the top executives get his hair cut. (It was a big deal because he hadn't cut it in ten years.) The CEO came back from a three-day party in San Diego with his hair dyed a different color. Finally, a wine shipment arrived mid-day. The CEO has his collection of red wines in his office. At four o'clock, he sent an e-mail around saying it was wine o'clock, and they all dropped everything to sample the latest shipment. I guess they are thinking of having a wine cellar built in the office. I can't wait to meet these people. They sound a little eccentric. Sounds like Tommy will have no trouble "conforming." He left today in his Doc Marten boots and earrings. He has an office and is filling it with his computer programming and management books as well as his personal effects. I guess they do work there. He had his first big interview last night.

It seemed like an easy week. Aleks is in a stage now where he can entertain himself for quite some time. I think I can actually do work while he is playing. I believe this is a very small window of time. He will be walking any day, and everything will change again!

Something is wrong with Creepy. We both noticed she is dropping weight at an amazingly fast rate. One day she was a fat cat. Now she is about normal. I think I will make a vet appointment. They are due for shots anyway. Poor Creepy. Maybe Aleks is just keeping her on the go.

I better go. As usual, I have about fourteen things to do while Aleks is napping. I smell my breakfast burning, and a shower would be a good thing.

Love, Stacey

Subject: sugar kitty
Date: Thu, 17 Feb 2000

We lucked out, and Creepy stabilized with the small amount of glucose we were giving her. She will not need to go in for weekly monitoring for now. That is a huge relief. It was going to set us back $400–$500 a month. Our other kitty lost a tooth. Now she is really funny looking. Time for kitty dentures.

Love, Stacey

Subject: hello from Seattle
Date: Sat, 25 Mar 2000

Hello,

We visited Tommy at work today. I now really believe this place Tommy calls work really exists. I met his coworkers. They all seem pretty nice. The offices are also nice. Each person had his/her space individually decorated. Many were very eclectic. Tommy's is very interesting. He took several of my bright paintings to hang.

Subject: trip to Wisconsin
Date: Tue, 28 Mar 2000

Well, we are booked. We might make a quick stop in Madison for some Whole Food yummies. You will see us between 3:00 and 4:00. Can't wait! I'm glad we will get to see everyone. We will stay in Boscobel until Wednesday morning.

I think I am going to join a health club today. The idea of doing it has seemed ridiculous considering that we have the equipment downstairs. There is a club by the market that has a daycare center. I've come to the conclusion that it's the only way I can manage to get a workout in. I think I am more concerned about what the daycare center is like than the workout facilities. Give me a rusty old weight machine and a good nanny, and I'll be happy! It seems expensive, but if I compute the costs, it is still less than I was paying Lisa to come once a week. If I give up my morning lattes, that will make up for most of it.

Love, Stacey

Subject: hello
Date: Thu, 6 Apr 2000

How's your week? Ours has been busy. Aleks has had some new experiences. His new nanny came on Tuesday. I guess the morning was a little rough, but after his nap, he snapped out of it and they had a good time. He was giving her kisses by the time I got home.

He was funny last night before bedtime. He had me read nearly every book on the bookshelf, but he avoided the *Goodnight Moon* book because he knows that's the book we read last, right before he goes to sleep. He is learning the art of procrastination especially when it comes to bedtime.

I filled out my census form finally. I couldn't decide whether Aleks spoke English not at all or not very well. Tommy thought not very well. I was also convinced that I should have said "yes" to having a condition lasting more than six months that affected my ability to learn, concentrate, or remember. That would be sleep deprivation. Sometimes I would also say it made it difficult to bathe or dress myself (the next question).

Love, Stacey

CHAPTER 6

December 14 is the Big Date

Subject: Hi from Seattle
Date: Fri, 5 May 2000

Had my ultrasound yesterday. It looks like Dec. 14th is the big date. I am about eight weeks along.

I am going to a retreat this weekend. Should be back sometime Sunday afternoon. The boys are planning all kinds of fun. Aleks is helping me type again stacey+

To: Stacey Reynolds
Sent: Sunday, August 20, 2000
Subject: Christmas

Hi, Stacey and Tommy,

I made those reservations. We will be in Seattle Christmas Day, arriving at 2:37 p.m. for a "low-key" Christmas. We will leave December 30.

Love, Mom

Subject: Re: Christmas
Date: Sun, 20 Aug 2000

Yay! I asked Tommy what he thought, and he said he would like it if you came for Christmas. It will be so nice to share it with family.

Good luck tomorrow at school. I hope you have good students this year.

Love, Stacey

Subject: hi from Seattle
Date: Sat, 14 Oct 2000

Hi, Mom and Gary,

We had a busy week. Tommy worked late every night.

Aleks and I stayed busy, too. I started some projects like sorting baby clothes. I have two grocery bags of clothes that look like they are unisex. I put 2 1/2 bags away as boy-only clothes. The nursery is cleaned out, and I have the changing table in there. I'd like to get a rocker if the room is big enough. I've also been working on Aleks' room. I bought a toy storage system at IKEA. I still haven't finished putting the shelves together, but his toys are now sorted in bins. The screw holes for the shelves weren't lining up. A project like that is fun to share with Aleks for about 10 minutes, and then it loses its luster as the screws run off around the house. Maybe Tommy or I can work on it this weekend.

Love, Stacey

Subject: Hi from Seattle
Date: Sat, 11 Nov 2000

Hi, Mom and Gary,

Salute to my favorite war veteran!! ! ! !

As this election thing presses on, I sincerely wish I would have taken my little sister's advice and voted for Nader. I am becoming more and more convinced that neither of these men is worthy of the task.

I only wish I could stay up late enough to see late night talk shows. It's really getting funny.

Love, Stacey

Subject: happy thanksgiving
Date: Wed, 22 Nov 2000

Hello, Mom and Gary,

I will probably talk to you tomorrow, but I thought I would update you on my doctor's appointment. Things are starting to happen. I am about 2 cm dilated and 70% effaced. She said I could go into labor anytime, or she (the baby) could hang around until my due date. I'm pretty excited, although we aren't really ready. You should see the nursery—what a mess! I need to find a quicker way to get to the hospital. It took me 45 minutes to get there this afternoon with the holiday traffic. Hopefully we won't go until later at night.

Stacey

Subject: still the same
Date: Wed, 29 Nov 2000

Hello,

I had my doctor's appointment today. No new news. I'm in about the same place as last week. Feeling good, though I'm getting lousy sleep. Doing crazy things like eating large pieces of chocolate cake and then cleaning the whole house. (That's what I did last night.)

Love, Stacey

Subject: hi from Seattle
Date: Tue. 5 Dec 2000

Hello,

Well I got my Christmas packages all sent and got dinner ordered for Christmas Day. Now when am I going to have this baby?

I hope our weather stays nice. It is sunny and 50 today. Aleks and I went to the zoo this morning. They have a baby elephant and gorilla there both around 6-8 weeks old. They are sooooo cute, it's enough to make a pregnant girl like me weepy.

Kassia Rose Lesiewicz was born December 15, 2000

Subject: Re: Snowy Monday
Date: Mon, 18 Dec 2000

Hi,

We look forward to seeing you. It will be nice to have a few extra hands around. Aleks will love the attention, too. We did get more sleep last night, which is good. Kassia is getting cuter all the time. Aleks seems to be doing well. He is a little sensitive though. He is adorable with her.

Love, Stacey

To: Stacey Reynolds
Sent: Thursday, December 21
Subject: How are things?

Hi,

Just a short note to tell you how much we have enjoyed the pictures of Kassia. She is beautiful.

Your mom brought over the lovely Christmas basket from you, and I want to tell you that we will enjoy the coffee and truffles very much. There's nothing like Seattle coffee and sweets!

Hope you are getting some sleep, Stacey. I know how frustrating it is to have the little one waking you up so often. Maybe Daddy and a bottle is going to be a good solution.

Love, Grandma Lois

Subject: Re: How are things?

Date: Thu, 21 Dec 2000

Hello, Grandma and Grandpa,

I'm glad you liked the basket. I also wanted to let you know we received the box you sent. I have been hiding the boxes in the basement. Aleks is very interested in what's inside.

Kassia has been sleeping as well as can be expected for a newborn. I try to take two short naps a day even if only 10 minutes. I think she is going to be sleepier than Aleks. Overall, she seems very content. We will send some more pictures soon. We took some cute ones of her and Aleks together. I am feeling very good. It was really an easy birth, which is amazing because of her size. We were only at the hospital three hours before she was born.

We are settling into a routine here at home. Tom has been a wonderful helper, and Aleks seems to be doing well. Now that I'm up and about, I am trying to set aside some dedicated alone time for him. He loves his dad, but I don't want him to feel like he lost his mommy!

I sure look forward to Mom and Gary's visit. I can't believe they will be here soon. It will make the holiday extra special. I hope you have a good Christmas. Tell everyone hello and drive carefully.

Love, Stacey

To: Stacey D. Reynolds
Sent: Thursday, December 21
Subject: Dollhouse

Hi, Stacey,

Yesterday Gary mailed Kassia's dollhouse. When it comes, don't try to lift it yourself. It's a very heavy package. We know she's much too little to play with it now, but I think it has to be put together and decorated inside, too. That should take a few years. Isn't she lucky to have an interior designer for a mother?

Mom

Subject: Re: Dollhouse
Date: Thu, 21 Dec 2000

A dollhouse, how cool! I especially like the fact that we can decorate it. Sounds like, a fun project for all of us. You might be here before the box. I can't wait! Please send your itinerary so Tommy can pick you up. Everything is going well here. Kassia is a sleepy girl except for between 2 and 3:30 a.m., when I have a hard time getting her back to sleep.

Our Christmas tree is coming down today. It looks like a Charlie Brown tree. It was to the point of looking pretty ugly if not a bit hazardous.

We did take one family picture in front of it yesterday. We will string the lights around the window and decorate the fireplace. Hopefully it will look a little bit like Christmas. I'm so glad you're coming. It will be fun!!!

Stacey

Date: Tue, 2 Jan 2001

It's been a challenging and interesting day. I failed my first day at home alone, and Tommy ended up coming home early. For good reason, I guess. First of all, I didn't sleep last night. Kassia was a hungry girl. I felt like I nursed all night long. Really, I didn't get any serious sleep in until 4:30. It's funny because I got a rocker thinking I could be really organized and strategic when she does wake up and get myself back in bed as quickly as possible and hopefully get her on a schedule. She had something else in mind. They say a growth spurt at about two weeks is not unusual, and this "cluster feeding" comes with it. Hopefully just one night.

Our New Year's was quiet. A little champagne and chocolate for a weary couple of parents!

Love, Stacey

Subject: one-month birthday
Date: Mon, 15 Jan 2001

Hi, Grandma and Grandpa,

Kassia is full of smiles today on her one-month birthday. It's going to be fun to see her react to things. She's sleeping in the sling now.

We went to Issaquah yesterday. Tom picked up some work. We stopped and had pizza, and we drove around and looked at the town. It's a pretty town—a little less suburban than I thought. Maybe we could live there some day.

We looked at a house yesterday in Seattle, too. It was in our neighborhood. I had my eye on it because it was cute, and it was on a nice street. What a shocker! It was small, needed tons and tons of work, and was priced at $409,000. I would be totally depressed living there until we sunk about $200,000 of work into it. Makes Issaquah and renting look pretty good. Or we could move back to the Midwest and buy a really nice house for half that.

Love, Stacey

Date: Wed, 17 Jan 2001

Hello,

Kassia has been taking her bottle. Tommy was thrilled that he was able to feed her. He doesn't know what he's getting into. I have about three hours of unused spa time! I'll probably wait on that, but maybe Tom and I could slip out for another quick dinner. That would be nice.

Love, Stacey

Subject: Hi from Seattle
Date: Thu, 8 Feb 2001

We had snow this morning! It barely covered the grass and is now melted.

It was Kassia's first snow here. Come to think of it, it was Aleks' too! He said, "Oh, oh," when he saw it on my coat.

Tom is showing our condo on Friday morning. They sound like good ones, I hope they like it.

I better go. I hear Kassia pooping, and I'm so hungry I can't believe it.

Love, Stacey

Subject: Re: Hi from Mom
Date: Wed, 21 Feb 2001

We are having a stressful week, but I think things will get better soon. Tom's work is slow, fortunately he is the human resources manager as well as recruiter, otherwise he'd be in trouble. I've been a little overwhelmed so it's nice to have him around a little more, but we could use the income. It looks like we might rent out the condo but the only people we've got want a 6-month lease beginning April 1. I think I need to do a feng shui over-haul around here. We seem to be doing fine in the kids category. They are just beautiful and sweet. I better go take advantage of this coffee buzz while it lasts.

Love Stacey

Subject: hello from Seattle
Date: Fri, 23 Feb 2001

hi Mom and Gary,

today we had an early morning photo session. kassia cried throughout. we may have gotten one or two good ones to pick from. i picked her up with my arm around her belly and made her spit up all over her cute little red dress. Most of the pictures will have her crying with a big wet splotch on her dress. a representative for one of the Mariner pitchers is looking at our condo tomorrow. tommy checked his stats on the net. sounds like a good rookie. we probably won't have to worry about his ability to pay the rent. we will be lucky if he takes it. only one week will go unrented. perfect. have to keep our fingers crossed.sunday we may look at houses.

Love Stacey

one handed typing

CHAPTER 7
"Shake-up"

Subject: EARTHQUAKE
Date: Fri, 2 Mar 2001

Hi, all,

I'm sure you've seen the repetitive coverage on our big quake and you already know that we are OK. I feel like I've either been too excited or too tired to convey our experience accurately. Here it is: I was having a bad morning. It was taking forever to get everyone ready for our toddler class at Seattle Community College. Aleks really wanted to go, so, I did my best to pull us together. I wore a funny scarf on my head because I just could not get my hair to look right. I had a weird feeling that day. Things were getting harder, not easier for us. At the same time, I had a feeling that there was going to be a "shake-up" and that things would get better soon.

We made it to class approximately one hour late. Aleks played with some airplanes while I swapped parenting stories with some of my friends in the class. Kassia bobbed in front of me in the kangaroo pack. Everyone was marveling at how quickly she's grown. Soon it was snack time. We washed the toddler's hands and sat them down at the miniature table and chairs around the room. Aleks had consumed about two mouthfuls of crackers when the shaking began.

This was my fourth or fifth earthquake since moving to the West Coast six years ago, so it didn't take me long to figure out what it was. I remember saying "earthquake" while looking at another wide-eyed mom across the table. The next thing I did was glance at the big windows about 10 feet away from us. I must have been thinking about tornados back in the Midwest because I instinctively wanted to move everyone away from that glass. I grabbed Aleks, and we ventured across the room. I remember it being a little difficult to walk, but I was walking and ducking to take cover at the same time. We tucked our heads under a toddler table on the other side of the room. My friend Jennifer was under there. She said, "Poor Lara," our friend whose labor was induced the night before. She was either in the middle of it or had a very new baby.

There was the usual earthquake dialog—"Oh, it's a big one," and "Is it over yet?" Nothing was falling in the room. It was designed with solid low shelves for children. The most unnerving thing was that the hard vinyl composite floor was rolling beneath us. When the shaking slowed, people began worrying about their homes and where their loved ones were. The toddlers were amazing. They had not made a peep and actually went back to their snacks. They definitely sensed something was wrong but were quick to get back to their old routine—a routine that was quickly broken up when we were told that class was over, and we had to leave.

I didn't know what to do next. I really had to go to the bathroom, had two children with me, a diaper bag, crackers, and water. I figured we would just go home but didn't know if traffic would be bad or if roads and bridges would be intact. I decided to take the freeway thinking the ship canal bridge would be best. Our trip home was absolutely uneventful. We had about four miles to drive, and traffic was moving just a little slow but no backups yet. I think everyone on the road was like me, not quite sure what was ahead, if the bridges would be closed and what not. No damage was apparent where I was driving. I had no sense of how big the quake was. I scanned through radio stations and actually only a couple had begun coverage. I laughed out loud when one of them broke into the song "I feel the earth move under my feet...." A good release of any tension I was holding in. I was about a half mile from home when the first real reports of damage were coming in. I knew then that it was a pretty big one.

I thought about Tom but knew he would be safe in his newer low-rise office building. I was glad he was no longer working on the 43rd floor downtown. The main thing I was worried about were the floating bridges. If something happened to them, he would not be able to reach us from the eastside where he works.

I pulled into our driveway and remembered to get out and smell for gas before letting the kids out. No gas, and a quick assessment of our basement showed minimal damage, just one broken vase. I brought the kids in and spent what seemed like the remainder of the day glued to the TV. I was relieved when Tom came home about 30 minutes later. He had a big grin on his face. He was enjoying this. He got to have an "earthquake day." The power was out at his office, and it looked like a war zone. Pictures fell off the wall. Planters fell over, and his computer monitor slid off his desk. He looked outside during the quake and saw waves in the sidewalk. After swapping stories, we decided to go out for lunch and a beer to soothe our rattled nerves. We went to a Mexican restaurant, which was busy with people who had an early end to their work day.

All in all, I never feared for our lives. Sometimes you feel like you tempt fate living out here. For example, 24 hours after the quake, we were scheduled to have pictures taken at Sears located in the Starbucks building you've seen on the news. Needless to say, they were cancelled. When you look at statistics most earthquakes are not that deadly of an event, at least with our modern structures. Don't get me wrong, I really don't want to be here when the shallow 8.0 hits.

Things were quickly back to normal for us. I think the TV news media has a way of making events like this look bigger than they are, though I know many lives have been disrupted. Love you all,

Stacey

Carole: Stacey's sister Laurie and husband Todd were expecting their first baby in the spring of 2001. Niece Remington would be born September 25 of that year.

Subject: Re: Baby
Date: Mon, 5 Mar 2001

Hi, Kids,

Laurie just called. She had her doctor's appointment today. She heard the baby's heartbeat, and it was "strong and fast." Everything is going fine. She was lying on the couch when she called tonight and said she didn't know if she had the energy to go back in her office and e-mail her sisters and brother like she promised to do after her doctor's appointment, so I said I'd do it for her. So, this is it.

Love, Mom

From: Stacey D. Reynolds

Thanks for the update. I'm happy all was well. I was going to call and then thought I'd check my e-mail to see if there was a message from Laurie. I was thinking about her! Hope your week is starting out good.

Love, Stacey

Subject: yucky week
Date: Fri, 16 Mar 2001

Hi, Mom and Gary,

What a week. I think Tom and I are in the Seattle "Survivor" series. It will be interesting to see which one of us cracks first.

We both started the week with a horrible flu. The worst I've ever had. On Wednesday one-third of Tom's company was laid off. He had to give up his vacation week and go in to pick up the pieces. Kassia's skin problem got worse. She is itchy at night and has been waking nearly hourly for a week now. I took her to the naturopathic doctor yesterday. My diet has been implicated. A restrictive diet has been recommended until we figure it out. To be eliminated: dairy, eggs, wheat, chocolate, coffee, alcohol, peanuts, corn, citrus, spicy foods, greasy foods. What's left??????????

On the bright side, Kassia did not get the flu, and Tom did not get laid off. He has a job—at least this month. He has two other good jobs already lined up (impressive!). It looks like we have renters for April 1. We may sell anyway and walk away with more money than we ever thought, a nice down-payment on one of the modest $500,000 homes we've seen???? My new diet will be very slimming. Nursing moms need 2,000 calories per day. Easy to do with chocolate and Ben and Jerry's. Hard to do with rice cakes and leafy greens.

Luv, Stacey

Subject: a note from Stacey
Date: Tue, 20 Mar 2001

Mom and Gary,

The week is starting out better than last. We have beautiful spring weather after some much-needed rain. We just went to the post office and I saw hyacinths, daffodils, tulips, azaleas, and cherry blossoms. It's nice to be in a neighborhood where you can walk and see these things.

Tom is talking to someone about a job today. He's not confident his company is making payroll at the end of the month. Yikes!!!! It would be nice to have him closer to home. It sounds like more money, and perhaps he can get a little signing bonus to keep us out of a pinch.

He is also talking to a realtor who swears he can get $350K for our condo. Everyone else says $300-320K. Unless Tom totally hates him, we will probably have him do it. The market is slowing because of the stock market. Hopefully it won't sit too long.

Kassia's rash was progressively getting better... then a little backslide yesterday. I ate none of the foods on the forbidden list. Perhaps it's my imagination or a fluke. Basically, I'm encouraged. I hope we can narrow it down in the next week or two so I can get on a semi normal diet.

I think we slept better last night. The scary part is I don't remember. Either we slept well, or I am getting too comatose to even know.

Love, Stacey

Subject: the magic music box
Date: Thu, 5 Apr 2001

Hi, Mom and Gary,

Just wanted to let you know the little music box you got Kassia works like a gem. I trained her to associate it with falling asleep. I play it while I nurse her just before bed. If she wakes up before my designated time, I press that little remote before she fully wakes up and back to sleep she goes. Tommy almost threw it out the window the first night when I had to play it 10–15 times. The second night only three times, and then last night only two and she slept for six hours straight! Yay!

Date: Tue, 10 Apr 2001

Hi, Mom,

Kassia's rash got pretty bad again. I had to get the "big guns" out again—the antibiotic cream and cortisone. I'm more baffled as to what it can be. I'm trying to give up coffee and chocolate, now thinking maybe it's something that builds up in her system and her skin shows a response after it reaches a certain level. Just my theory. The diet and all these things are actually quite healthy and, believe it or not, I do find a lot to eat. I just have to be more creative and it requires more prep than I like. Once in a while I go crazy and just have to cheat.

Needless to say, Kassia has not slept well the last couple of nights. She was quite itchy.

The biggest news is that I booked flights for June. We will be staying in Boscobel the 12–17. Can't wait. I miss everyone so much. It looks like we will probably stay at the Super 8. Tommy insists this time. The four of us will be a three-ring circus and will overtake anyone's home. I hope we don't insult anyone—we always enjoy staying with you. You make us feel right at home!

It's rainy and cool today. Aleks and I planted some pansies in back in spite of the weather. It is one of those days when he has more energy than the walls of this house can handle. Kassia spit up on the keyboard, and I think Aleks is pooping his pants. Back to my mom duties.

Love and kisses, Stacey

Subject: happy Easter
Date: Sat, 14 Apr 2001

Hi, everyone,

Hope you had a nice visit today. Wish we could've been there.

Aleks was successful at the egg hunt. He passed up a number of eggs for the chocolate treats laying around. He walked away with five miniature Hershey bars, 13 chocolate Kisses, and two Reese's bars. Later I found him with chocolatey hands and mustache. Kassia just took it all in. She can't wait until next year. After the egg hunt, we went up to the tulip fest. It was nice, but traffic was bad. Aleks enjoyed seeing tractors, cows, sheep, and horses—especially the tractors. Just wait until he goes back to the Midwest.

This is sad. For some reason, he had the impression we were going to Grandma and Grandpa's house. I think it had something to do with seeing a lot of airplanes. He was upset on the way home because it was obvious that wasn't in the plan. Poor little guy. Oh, by the way, we will take you up on the invitation to stay in June. Are you sure five days isn't too much? The kids are adorable, but Aleks can sometimes be every bit of a 2-year-old, and Kassia has a loud cry. Gotta go.

Love you all, Stacey

Subject: Re: more pictures
Date: Wed, 18 Apr 2001

Hi, Mom and Gary,

I'm glad you enjoyed the pictures. We had our individual Sears pictures taken on Monday, finally. Guess what? Kassia started to cry and cry. We did get one photo that turned out. It is a silly one with Tigger the tiger. It was sort of a joke, but now it is the only one I've got. She looks a little like Lesley's baby photos in it. We went back to the Sears in the damaged Starbuck's building. That was the first time I'd been down in that part of the city since the quake. I was amazed at the number of buildings undergoing repairs. I visited my old coworkers also while down there. That building had a lot of cosmetic damage and was yellow tagged by the city. They can still run business out of it while repairs are being done. Glad I wasn't there.

We went to Seattle Central Community College today for class. As usual, Aleks would have nothing to do with the music circle. He found a secret stash of whales and sharks under the sink and played with them most of the time. Tommy and I are thinking of going to the "radical mamas and pa-pas potluck tonight." We don't exactly know who these people are, but we've been invited. I'm trying to decide if I should wear my chains or tie dye. It sounds like a good way to meet people, though. Tommy had a fender bender today. No one hurt, but the Geo is in need of repairs. Yuk.

There is a glut of condos for sale in our building. More than the realtor has ever seen. It will probably take longer to sell our place than hoped, but so far, no price reductions. It's only been on the market 20 days. I won't start freaking until it goes over two months.

I was reaching up in the cupboard to get some rice cakes today, and a bag of chocolate chips showered upon me. I had to pick them all up without eating any. This diet is getting old.

Love, Stacey

Subject: CELL PHONES BLESSING OR CURSE?
Date: Sat, 19 May 2001

Hi, Mom and Gary,

Tommy and I had a date night last night. We dropped the kids off at the health club. Kassia was stuffed to the brim with cereal, and Aleks was ready to play with trains. We left the childcare center my recently acquired cell phone number—just in case. Our first stop was the Crocodile Café, one of our old favorites. As we walked, we felt this enormous sense of freedom that we haven't experienced in a while. We ordered some drinks. I took two sips of my Newcastle Nut Brown Ale and was leaning back in the booth enjoying the artwork that was surrounding me then RIIIIIIIIIIIING! The cell phone went off. Kassia was crying like crazy in the background, and they couldn't calm her. Tommy went up and settled our tab, and we went back down the hill to the health club. The poor little girl was just gasping when she saw us but settled down quickly. She went to sleep in about 10 minutes.

We decided to give it a second try since we were going to have to pay for the childcare services regardless. We made it to the swanky restaurant where we had reservations. The place has great food and is totally romantic: candlelit tables, jazz, waiters in white, the whole works. We ordered wine and were having a nice conversation while I finished my salad when RIIING! I answered and could hear Kassia in the background again. I left Tommy at the table with the wine and our soon-to-be-arriving dinner and dashed back to the club. I just picked her up, and she stopped crying. I wasn't going to try again, so we just sat and waited for Tommy to come back with our $60 dinner in cardboard boxes. We went home. Aleks went right to bed. I was having trouble getting Kassia settled, so we decided to dig into our cold dinner with her bouncing on our laps. We were about half-done when she blasted the biggest poo. I'm sure that was the source of some of her grief. Tommy was just about going crazy at this point. I suggested he go and get us some dessert while I cleaned up Kassia and put her to sleep. It worked. We were able to have a romantic dessert.

It sounds like it was miserable, but actually we had fun. It was kind of funny.

I don't know if I like these cell phones. I will forward the numbers to you. I don't plan on using mine except for emergencies. Have a diaper to change. I'll talk to you soon.

Love, Stacey

Subject: ready to go
Date: Sat, 9 Jun 2001

I was putting Aleks down for his nap and he was begging for one of the goodies I bought for the plane. I told him he had to wait until we went on the airplane. A few minutes later, he was calling me and saying "Aleks ready to go airplane." I peeked in his room and he had his little suitcase packed with whale books and his tippy cup. Can't wait to see you. Kassia is ready to charm you with her silly babble.

Love, Stacey

Subject: Re: Hi from Mom
Date: Thu, 2 Aug 2001

Hi, Mom and Gary,

Kassia's appointment did not go so great. She is really allergic to a lot of things. Mostly food now. She is starting to become allergic to cats. They said she would likely grow out of all the allergies except for the peanuts. It's pretty complicated with the diet adjustments we will need to make, but certainly there are worse things to have happen. They gave me an antihistamine to give her at night. I don't like to give it to her, but her skin seemed to clear up immediately. Better go get my sleep.

I just can't wait for next week!

Love, Stacey

Subject: working girl again
Date: Wed, 29 Aug 2001

Hi, Mom and Gary,

Guess what? I start work again on Friday. Yep, I may be working anywhere from 10—20 hours per week. Yikes!

I currently only have a sitter for Fridays. But I may luck out. The woman who is leaving EHC to go back to school was formerly a nanny. I asked if she would like to sit for Aleks and Kassia about 20 hours per week around her school schedule. It sounds like she wants to do it. It will be perfect if I can have someone I trust, and I will also do the majority of the work from home, so I can go upstairs and give them kisses whenever I want. This couldn't be timelier because Tommy's company is really having troubles. They announced yesterday they would not be making payroll. Not too many people showed up today. Poor Tommy is still working his butt off, though. He also has his feelers out. It's a little scary, but I'm sure he won't be unemployed for long. We'll see what happens....

Love, Stacey

Subject: car seat
Date: Tue, 11 Sep 2001

Hi, Mom and Gary,

We got the car seat today. Thanks! That will really help out. Can't write much now. What a day...

Love, Stacey

To: Stacey D. Reynolds
Sent: Wednesday, September 12, 2001
Subject: Re: car seat

Hi, Stacey,

Yes, it was "quite a day" yesterday. I wish you would move to a smaller city away from the Canadian border.

I worked today subbing for the art teacher. It went really well. Hope the next two days are the same.

Love, Mom

Subject: Re: car seat
Date: Wed, 12 Sep 2001

I thought that you were probably subbing. I'm sure it is nice to walk to work.

Yes, I would have slept better last night if I was nestled in the hills of southwest Wisconsin instead of hanging off the coast with military planes flying overhead. But there were definitely worse places to be. I'm going to try to get some good sleep tonight.

You know when I said I was dizzy the other morning? I realized I had slept five hours uninterrupted for the first time in three years that night. It's getting better.

Stacey

Subject: a note from Stacey
Date: Sat, 29 Sep 2001

Everything is back to normal after our trip. Kassia slept through last night which was good. They were kind of screwed up after switching time zones and then with the daylight savings ending.

Love Stacey

P.S. attached are a couple of things I wrote about our plane trip

Flying in these times:

When we got to the airport a full two hours early, we found that 25% of the parking garage was blocked off for security reasons. We were able to find a spot easily but at the end of our trip we found that parking rates had been increased to $20/day.

The armed National Guards caught Aleks' eye. They did not seem strange to me because it reminded me of just about any other country I had been to. I did not think they looked mean enough. They were chatting and laughing. A sign in Minneapolis offered them free cookies. No wonder they were so happy.

The security line in Seattle was minimal, but in Madison we waited at least 30 minutes to get through. Before our plane took off in Minneapolis, the pilot made a general announcement asking passengers to be extra aware of any suspicious activity on the plane and to notify them if we see anything. Just when I thought airline service had reached an all-time low, on our return flight, I overheard the flight attendant scolding a passenger for asking for sugar for his coffee. "Because of recent events, we do not offer cream or sugar on our flights. In fact, you are lucky you get a meal. Most airlines are not even serving food." Our dinner consisted of a sandwich, a small bag of carrots, a cookie, and water. Before taking off in Minneapolis, the flight attendant came over to me and reminded me that I was prohibited from using baby powder on the flight.

Bring a book. There were no headphones or movies. In fact, all the video equipment had been removed from this DC-10. The safety film was flashed on a wall over the bulkhead seats without the screen. I heard the flight attendant explaining this to a passenger. If they are cutting back on complimentary headphones to save money, I don't even want to know what other corners they are cutting.

Subject: RE: Hi
Date: Tue, 2 Nov. 2001

Hi,

We had a fun Halloween. Aleks changed his mind and wanted to be a bat at the last minute. We talked him back into being a firefighter because I couldn't figure out how to make wings "on the fly." Kassia wore her striped tiger shirt and leggings. She wouldn't let me paint whiskers and I couldn't find the little cat nose, so she wore a zebra thing on her head, at least for the pictures. Poor little baby.... her first Halloween, and I guess she was a "zigger." We went to the Wallingford Center where they handed out candy at the stores.

Today we went to Bainbridge on the ferry. I had to measure a job there. It's nice we could make an outing of it. Yes, I'm really busy. I think I will have 20 hours in this week.

Stacey

Subject: Hi from Seattle
Date: Wed, 3 Nov. 2001

Hi, everyone,

Tom and I have made the decision not to do Christmas presents this year. We thought we would prefer to spend the time with family and therefore will spend the money to fly back, etc. Please do not purchase gifts for us. Of course, you can buy gifts for the kids. We want to make their Christmas as special as possible. If anyone objects to this, I have some fabulous fruitcakes leftover from last year I can send you. Just kidding. If all goes well, we will see you on the 15th!

Love, Stacey

CHAPTER 8
Help from the Midwest

In late November 2001, Stacey's sister Lesley and her husband, Jon, rejecting their "yuppie" lifestyle, left their jobs in Chicago, sold their Volkswagen Jetta and headed for Seattle. They would live in the lower level of the house Stacey and Tommy rented in the Wallingford district. Lesley would be Stacey's new nanny, and Jon hoped to find his dream job as a bike messenger.

Subject: bike
Date: Mon, 12 Nov 2001

Lesley and Jon,

Arrived today in Seattle... one bike in a Bianchi box. Stored safely in our garage. Looking forward to those gourmet meals, Jon. I'm tired of take-out Indian food. See you soon.

Love, Stacey

Subject: potty training
Date: Wed, 14 Nov 2001

Grandkid report:

Aleks has been wearing undies all week. So far, no accidents. YEAH! Kassia is getting two new teeth on top for a total of six.

Mom and Dad are doing fine. We seem to be balancing our responsibilities a little better this week. Tommy got some promising news on his employment today. We also saw a thing in the paper about calling the bank if you have been laid off. They are more than willing to work out deals on your loan payments. They are bending backwards for laid-off tech workers to keep their business. We haven't had troubles yet, but we might work something out, so we don't go too far into debt. Looking forward to the arrival of Lesley and Jon.

Love, Stacey

Subject: hello
Date: Wed, 28 Nov 2001
From: Jon and Lesley

Hi, Mom and Gary!

Everything is going pretty well in Seattle so far. Jon is still looking for a job. He put in 3 or 4 applications on Monday at bike messenger places. One or two of them were actually looking for people and the others just said they were always taking applications. Hopefully something comes up. He is going to give it a week before he starts looking for other things.

The kids are being really good for Aunt Lesley and Uncle Jon. It has been easy babysitting for them so far. Today was a big babysitting day. We watched them from 10 until 2:30, and we are watching them again tonight so Stacey and Tommy can go out on a date. Aleks and I made a "train" out of couch cushions this morning and one of the places we went was Grandma Carole's and Grandpa Gary's. I asked Aleks what was at your house and he said chookies (cookies) and Rover. When the train arrived at your house, he pretended to give you great big hugs and then he pretended he went to sleep on Rover. It was cute.

Jon and I have been wandering around Seattle a lot. We have been taking the buses and walking and riding our bikes. We are trying to find the perfect coffee shop hangout. So far it looks like it is going to be the Coffee Messiah.

Friday night we are going to a party/concert for the second Anniversary of the WTO protests. There is going to be food and some bands and a lot of art displays. Sounds like fun.

Talk to you soon, Lesley

Subject: hand, foot, and mouth
Date: Thu, 29 Nov 2001

Yikes! I think Kassia has it. She has bumps on her feet and is going to the doctor today. No wonder she has been so crabby lately.

I'm afraid if our lovely weather doesn't scare Jon and Lesley away, then diseases involving blisters on the hands and feet and babies crying in the middle of the night will.

Stacey

Subject: bumpy baby
Date: Thu, 29 Nov 2001

Hi, Mom and Gary,

The doctor thinks it is probably the hand, foot, and mouth thing. Not a thing to be done. Not serious at all. Kassia seemed perky tonight. The best mood I've seen her in all week.

Jon responded to an advertisement in the paper for a messenger job. It sounds like a small company looking for part-time help. I hope it works out.

Love, Stacey

Date: Wed, 12 Dec 2001

Hi, Mom and Gary,

Got the cheese today. Thank you! Tommy ate the summer sausage before any of us could get a hold of it. He said he needed a little bit of meat before his interview today. He left today in his "monkey suit." He looked so handsome. If he does get the job and accepts it, he will probably have to forgo the blue hair for a while.

Lesley is doing such a nice job with Aleks and Kassia. They just love her. It is really nice to have them here.

Love, Stacey

"Stacey D. Reynolds" wrote:

Hi, Mom and Gary,

The kids are sick. Aleks was barfing all night long. Kassia actually slept through the night, AMAZING! But when I went in this morning, I discovered she had been sick also. I think they are both on the mend.

The big excitement in our neighborhood is that the Olympic torch will be going down 45th, just one block from our house tonight at 6:30. If it was anywhere else, I probably wouldn't go out of my way to see it, but it would be a nice time to take the kids out and get everyone some fresh air. Hope all is well there.

Love, Stacey

Subject: RE: hi from Seattle
Date: Thu, 24 Jan 2002

Aleks and I stood and waited for the torch to arrive for 45 minutes last night. Aleks said "maybe it is a late torch." Indeed, it was. I had him bundled up really well for the cold and wind, but I was not dressed adequately. We almost left early but Aleks really wanted to see it. It was exciting when it did arrive. Aleks got a little flag, and there were many cops on motorcycles, a helicopter right over our heads, and of course the torch.

Love, Stacey

Subject: Hi from Seattle
Date: Sat, 9 Feb 2002

Hello,

We finally got a good night of sleep! The night before last was totally crazy. Kassia slept until 4 a.m. but at 1:30 a.m. one of the kid's toys started "going off." Tom and I were wandering around the house searching for the source of something saying "star" and then playing the tune of "Row, Row, Row Your Boat." Was it the toy dragon? The Barney lap top? No... it was the toy phone wedged between Aleks' bed and the wall. After, that Tom and I both suffered from a bout of insomnia. I was sneezy and had to take Benadryl before I could get back to sleep. Tommy said he got back to sleep about three. The kids were both ready to get up at about 5:50. Talk to you soon.

Stacey

Jon and Lesley plan a cross-country biking adventure and a move back to the Midwest.

Subject: greetings from the slacker house
Date: Wed, 27 Mar 2002

Hi there,

Just put Aleks down for his nap. I think Kassia is waking up. Didn't time that one right, did I?

Tommy has a job interview on Friday. He left a message for me. I think it is one he is excited about. Things aren't looking good for his former company.

Lesley and Jon have been making all of their arrangements. I think they are getting excited. We will have to send a video of their departure either from our house or from the ferry dock and send it to you. It will be sad, but I am excited for them. Gotta go, Stacey

Subject: pictures
Date: Tue, 2 Apr 2002

Hi, everyone,

Hope you all had a good Easter. I heard you had quite a dinner! Our Easter was quiet. We did not leave the house. I made some bread in the bread machine and some fruit salad. Later in the day we grilled some veggie burgers outside. We had a pretty decent day.

I wanted to let you all know I sent some pictures along with a box of clothing that was sent to Laurie. They are Kassia's one-year pictures. Laurie may have told you my little story about leaving the pictures on top of the car after picking them up at the photographer. I got home and realized what I had done. I went back and re-traced my route just as it started to rain. I was lucky to find them about half way into my trip. The envelope was in very bad shape but fortunately the photos came through OK. A few of them have dimples from someone's studded tires.

Love, Stacey

Subject: RE: pictures
Date: Wed, 3 Apr 2002

Hi, Mom,

The kids continued to be a little sick today. Aleks threw up last night and for the first half of today. Suddenly he perked up just before dinner. He decided he wanted to eat and had very specific requests; he wanted two graham crackers and one bowl of Gorilla Munch cereal plain and one bowl of Gorilla Munch cereal with rice milk. I'm glad he is well. He ramped up to his usual full intensity by the end of the night. Kassia has just been a little feverish and cranky. She has developed this awful sounding screech, I hope that is temporary.

Tommy has three prospects now with possible second interviews. He goes in for the second time with a company tomorrow. It is looking good so far.

As far as a send-off for Jon and Lesley, I suggested a pancake breakfast. They are leaving very early in the morning, so perhaps we will need to do something the night before. I hope to take a little video of them if it is light enough outside. Weather is super nice here.

Stacey

CHAPTER 9

A Cross-Country Biking Adventure

Subject: Re: from MOM
Date: Wed, 03 Apr 2002
From: Jon and Lesley

Hi,

I'll email you our route, maybe tomorrow or Friday. I'll also call you with the cell phone number.

Jon rigged up a little solar panel for the back rack of his bike. We are going to use it to charge our cell phone and our rechargeable batteries. We tested it out, and it works! It only takes a few hours to charge the cell phone up in the sun, probably a little longer when it's not so sunny. The good thing about this is now we will probably be able to keep our cell phone on all the time since we won't have to worry about how we are going to charge it.

It looks like we will be staying in either campgrounds or state parks for the first five nights, but one night we may stay in a hostel. We'll just have to see how we're feeling.

Oregon and Northern California are going to be a breeze—there are campgrounds every 10 or so miles down the coast. Again, I'll email you the entire route, so you have an idea of which direction we're heading.

The weather is gorgeous here. Low 60's and sunny. It's very springy with all of the flowers, blossoms, and leaves on the trees. Jon was wishing he was out being a bike messenger today. He didn't get any nice weather like this when he was working. Ah, well, I told him he has plenty of nice sunny biking days ahead of him. I'll call you sometime soon. Tell everyone hi.

Love, Lesley

Subject: bike trip
Date: Fri, 05 Apr 2002
From: Jon and Lesley

Hi, Everyone,

As you probably know, we will be heading out on our big bike trip this Sunday, April 7th. Our trip will be about 4,400 miles. We don't have a set schedule as far as when we're going to be arriving at certain destinations. The best estimate we can come up with as far as how long our total trip is going to take is 3-6 months. We are taking our time, and if there are days we don't feel like riding, we won't. Also, if we find someplace we really like we may stay there for a few days. We will probably be camping almost all of the time, but we will stay in motels or hostels on occasion.

We are each bringing about 50 lbs. of gear. Lesley will carry stuff in the front and back panniers of her bike, and Jon is going to pull a bike trailer behind his bike. Some of the things we will be bringing are: tent, sleeping bags, sleeping rolls, cook stove, solar shower, tools, bike parts, clothes, books, cell phone, camera, first aid, water containers, and maps.

We will try to send out letters and pictures to keep ya'll updated on our journey. Use our cell phone number if you would like to contact us.

See you sometime this summer/early fall!

Love, Jon and Lesley

Date: Sun, 07 Apr 2002

Today's the big day! It's exciting and a little bit scary. I did make sure I took the time to appreciate my nice warm bed last night, though. Take care. We'll talk to you soon!

Love, Lesley and Jon

Subject: hi from Seattle
Date: Wed, 10 Apr 2002

Hi, Mom and Gary,

Just put the kids down for their afternoon nap. Yes, they both went down at the same time. Aleks is still mumbling something. He will do anything to delay his nap/bed time. How about if I brush my teeth? No, two "Sponge Bob Square Pants" episodes. What a little negotiator.

Tom got a job offer on Monday and may have another one tomorrow. He will have to make a decision between the two by end of week. They are both located on the Eastside. The pay after a year should be more than his previous job with the potential to make much, much more. I am so impressed at how quickly he worked that all out. He is nervous and excited. He suffered from a killer head ache starting on Monday. I think it is getting better.

I went in to work today. The showroom remodel I worked on is well underway and looks fantastic. I haven't been selling many cabinets, which is a bit of a problem. Maybe if the economy is picking up a little, it will help.

I think about Jon and Lesley all the time, every time the weather changes, every morning when we wake up, every time I see a bicyclist, and every night when we are making dinner. I bet they are having a wonderful time! I'm glad they are keeping in touch. It's fun to visualize where they might be. We were joking about hopping in the car and meeting up with them. They left their little camping espresso maker. We could deliver that to them.

We are going to stay put for the summer. We are going to stay in this house and not attempt to sell the condo at least until the fall. It will be nice to relax and just enjoy and do some camping and hiking with the kids. You can count on having a place to stay in the Wallingford neighborhood of Seattle should you decide to come out this way. Aleks would be very happy. We will plan to come to Boscobel around August 8. We would like to stay long enough to see Jon and Lesley, but we won't know their schedule until we get to that point.

Love, Stacey

Subject: map
Date: Wed, 10 Apr 2002

Did you plot out Lesley and Jon's route on a map? Lesley said you might have. I was wondering if it was in a format you could send me.... I think it would be a good lesson for Aleks to show him where they are at, etc. He keeps mentioning them. "Maybe Aunt Lesley will babysit me." I don't know if it has really hit him yet. Thanks, if you do send it.

Stacey

CHAPTER 10

Big Changes on the Horizon

Subject: thinking of you
Date: Tue, 14 May 2002

Hi, Mom,

I thought about you a lot on Mother's Day. I hope by now you got your envelope.

We had absolutely beautiful weather. It was 80 degrees. That is so out of the norm. Of course, on Monday, it was back to 55 and drizzle. We ended up barbequing chicken and sweet potatoes on the grill. I did a lot of gardening. That made me think of you, I think that I get my love of gardening from Mom. I've got my vegetable garden full. We are harvesting greens now. I am now starting to collect containers of stuff I don't have room for.

We finally got Tommy's motorcycle insurance and registration updated so he can ride. He has been riding to work when he can because he can get home through traffic faster. Yikes.

Tommy works late tomorrow night, and I have a meeting on Thursday night. I've had tons of billable hours, so that is great. Tommy got his first check on Friday. I feel like we are finally in a recovery mode. It is nice.

Stacey

Subject: hi from Seattle
Date: Mon, 3 Jun 2002

Hi, Mom and Gary,

We are so happy to have you coming out here—once again for the summer solstice. This time we can walk down to Fremont and see those nude bicyclists in the parade. Whooowee!!!!!!!

We had a big weekend. I didn't have to work (after working 15 hours last week), and the weather was nice, so we decided to go somewhere. We called a place on the coast and got a room and headed out about 10:30 am Saturday.

We got to the little town of Westport about 2:00. The motel was clean but quaint. It actually had a little kitchenette and a separate bedroom. Both good things with the kids. We ate at a Mexican restaurant, but I had to get my food to go because Kassia was restless and we couldn't verify through the broken English whether or not she could eat the food. Next, we went down to the ocean. It was like the Washington coast is 360 days of the year—cold, gray, windy, but wonderful if you have three layers of fleece and a good hat. Kassia would have none of it. I had to take her back to the car. Aleks and Tommy played a little bit. Aleks was raking with his rake. There's an endless amount of things you can rake on the beach, I guess. When he got back in the car, he said he never wanted to go back there again. It was too cold.

Back at the motel, we watched as much Cartoon Network as we could stand. Aleks said the motel and the TV were his favorite part. He is a carbon copy of his dad, I am sure.

The next day was warmer, so we DID go to the ocean again, this time to fly Aleks' kite. Kassia fell asleep in the car on the way, so she did not get to enjoy it. After that, Aleks and I found about six perfect sand dollars. Aleks wanted to throw them in the water, so we went down to the surf and threw them in.

It was sunny and warmer in Seattle when we arrived early Sunday afternoon.

Love, Stacey

Subject: Pooped in Seattle
Date: Tue, 25 Jun 2002

Hi, Mom and Gary,

Glad you are home safe. Aleks was a little sensitive today. Missing G & G, I think. Doctor's appointment went fine. They would have done another ultrasound, but I didn't want it. Some people think they aren't totally safe. Best not to have them done just for the fun of it. I may have one at 13 weeks; otherwise, not until 18 (I'm about 8.5 weeks now.)

"Stacey D. Reynolds" wrote:

Hi, Mom and Gary,

We are doing fine here. I've been feeling OK. I found out I was slightly anemic, so I am taking iron now. That usually doesn't hit until the second trimester, but it is good to know now so I can nip it in the bud. I hope to have all my energy back in a couple of weeks. We will see. Kassia went in for her 18-month check. She is doing fine. Her doctor was trying to think of ways to fatten her up. The only thing she came up with that Kassia wasn't allergic to was bacon.

Aleks' school was closed this week, so we have been entertaining ourselves at home. That little guy can play and play. Last night, he was Batman, Superman, and a bald eagle all wrapped up in one. Have a fun 4th.

Love, Stacey

Subject: those kids
Date: Tue, 9 Jul 2002

Mom and Gary,

Why is it that I can never find a pair of clean underwear for Aleks to wear and then he comes prancing out of the bedroom so proud of the way he has dressed himself—with three pairs of underwear on?

Kassia has been insisting on sleeping in her shoes or boots. Last night she slept in her sneakers.

I talked to our tenant yesterday, and it looks like he wants to sign another lease. That is good news. We want him to stay as long as possible because it is a lousy time to rent/sell. The prospect of staying in this house for another year is a lot better than moving back to the condo, especially now. So, I think we will stay put. I better get some work done. I've got a couple of new projects to bid on.

Love, Stacey

Subject: boy oh boy
Date: Fri, 16 Aug 2002

Hi, everyone,

Ultrasound and amnio went fine today. We have another active little baby—both doctors thought so. By now, you've guessed the big news. We are expecting another little boy. Kassia will retain her position as family princess. I'm taking it easy tonight. We ordered Thai food, and Tommy is feeding the kids. I'll probably talk to some of you this weekend. We will probably relax around the house except for seeing some big clipper ships on Lake Union. Hope all is well there.

Stacey

Date: Tue, 27 Aug 2002

Hi, Mom,

It has been a busy week of work for both of us. I am much too busy. I worked 16 hours this week, and I am heading for that many this week. It doesn't sound like much, but it is oh so hard to get those hours in without help. I had an emergency yesterday and needed to have plans done for an architect who was leaving town. I put in about five hours in three-minute intervals. My brain was mush by the end of the day. I have a meeting with my boss tomorrow to discuss options for the future. I don't think I can keep doing what I am doing presently for more than a couple of weeks without more help.

Stacey

Subject: RE: School Daze
Date: Mon, 9 Sep 2002

Hi, Mom,

Aleks did just fine today. It was such a cool place! It was a large brightly painted space with all kinds of play areas. They had giant firetrucks, bins of plastic animals (whales, sharks, dinosaurs, etc.), a train set, a little grocery store, a house to play in, puppet theaters, climbing structures, a library, and activity tables with art projects and Play-Doh.

On Wednesday I help with the class. I am scheduled to work in the house/store area, so I will play with the kids there at the appropriate times. There is a lot of work involved, but I think it is really a good thing, when you figure some pre-schools in Seattle run $6,000–$10,000 a year. It's nice that parents can contribute and, more or less, keep the school operating, be involved in what their kids are doing/learning, and learn some things themselves!

Ooh, a little kick from (jertzy, Ian, Kia)!!!!! We need to work on these names a little.

Stacey

To: Stacey D. Reynolds
Subject: Hi from Mom

Hi, Stacey,

You must be really busy since Aleks started school. I haven't heard from you. How is the pre-school teaching going?

I found a cute Polish boy's name in a name book—Koby. It is the familiar of Jacob.

Love, Mom

Subject: RE: Hi from Mom
Date: Tue, 17 Sep 2002

Mom,

Nice to hear from you. I am tired and busy, but Aleks' school is a blast. I hope my schedule evens out a little when the new sitter starts next week. Once she starts, I will be working M-W-F afternoons and hopefully not too much more.

Aleks asked me how babies come out yesterday... eek! Kassia took her first big kerplunk out of the crib today. She fell atop Aleks' red fire helmet and broke it. Aleks told me maybe we need to get a new red helmet and a new black helmet now. Only Aleks would negotiate a way to get two new helmets out of the deal.

Stacey

Date: Sat, 5 Oct 2002

Hi, Mom and Gary,

Tommy had a very good week at work. The seminar he put together was very successful and he got a call from a very good prospect who wants to meet with him.

Our week at school was fun. I was in charge of the art table on Wednesday and had to help eight eager three-year-olds string dinosaurs and straws to make dinosaur necklaces. It was the most popular spot to be. Everyone just had to have one! They used plastic needles to string the yarn through. Some kids caught on right away, others needed a lot of assistance. I did my best to help them all but let others just do it their own way. There were some funky looking necklaces. I don't know how you do it....

Stacey

Subject: boo boo face
Date: Wed, 16 Oct 2002

Hi, Everyone,

Lots of firsts yesterday for Aleks. I heard him count well into his twenties for the first time and recite the spelling of his name. And he got his first stitches! They weren't really stitches because now they have all these wonderful super glue techniques. He split his chin falling while climbing on a chair.

I'm getting big. I feel like I am about a month ahead of my other pregnancies. Lots of kicks now.

I painted Aleks' room, and the new bedding arrived for Kassia yesterday. It will be interesting to see how they like sharing a room. I wonder how they will ever get any sleep.

Stacey

Subject: baby update
Date: Thu, 17 Oct 2002

Had a doctor's appointment today and everything is going well. They did not say anything about my weight gain this time!

I scored big time on baby clothes. Someone in the co-op preschool has a little guy who is eight weeks old and has just outgrown all his 0–3 stuff. She gave me a garbage bag full of T-shirts, onesies, cute outfits, diapers, socks, and hats. Our little guy has all he needs for his first couple of months. Isn't that cool? I will probably give the co-op some money for it because it was supposed to go to the rummage sale fundraiser.

Got costumes today. When I asked Kassia what she wanted to be, she said "pumpkin" and pointed to her head. She then said, "big purple man," and "wings fly." I couldn't figure out what she wanted to be from that description. She obviously got some ideas when shopping for costumes with daddy this weekend. Anyway, she fell in love with a pink unicorn costume. I guess she got her wings at least. It is a darling costume. Aleks will be a firefighter once again this year. Actually, he wears his firefighter costume pretty much every day now—to school, to the store, to the library.

Stacey

Subject: doctor's appointment
Date: Tue, 12 Nov 2002

Hello,

Everything is looking and sounding good. I need to schedule an ultrasound as expected. That should be really cool, assuming that everything looks good. I have never had one this far along before.

Aleks saw a moving truck as we were driving today. He was asking what it did. I explained and then asked if he would want to move some day. He thought about it and said he would like to move by Grandma and Grandpa, then he could see you lots of times, and we would not have to buy plane tickets every time we go. Smart guy, huh? Maybe we should listen to him.

He also asked some difficult questions today about dying. He said he was sad because some people in a neighborhood died on the news. He's been very thoughtful lately. It keeps me on my toes and keeps the adult TV programs off for the most part.

Gotta get these kids down for their nap so I can have a little one myself.

Stacey

Subject: hi from Seattle
Date: Wed, 20 Nov 2002

Hi, Mom and Gary,

It's been a busy week here in Seattle. I actually think that I am doing too much and need to slow down. I have found myself literally running between things this week. Little Koby gets all shook up!

I sold two projects for work in the past couple of weeks. One is cabinets for a Belltown condo. It's a small but very complicated project for a young couple. The other is a huge $36,000 cabinet project on the East Coast for someone who works for Microsoft. In addition to making sure these projects go well, I have to start training people to take my place when I am off.

The extra money for all this work is good, and I don't feel exhausted, but this feeling of constantly being on the go and jumping from one thing to the next is what's bugging me. Today at 1:30, I was changing a diaper—at 2:00, I was downtown meeting with a contractor. It's crazy.

Our night life has been picking up, too. On Sunday, I went to a fancy cocktail party that someone from the pre-school held. I didn't know it was going to be such a fancy party and wore a sweater and jeans. I really had fun, even though I felt under dressed. It was one of those parties where they had goods to buy. She had a guy there who was selling designer handbags and jewelry. I can never leave those parties without buying something. Remember when I was in high school and bought all those cosmetics and facial cleansers and later returned them?

Anyway, I bought a necklace. Tommy is off the hook for my Christmas present. It seemed like an indulgence, but I love it and am glad I got it.

Last night Tommy and I had a date night. We saw the Michael Moore movie *"Bowling for Columbine."* I know Gary just loves that guy (ha, ha). The film's topic was gun control in the U.S. He took the usual stabs at big business, the media, politicians, and the NRA. It alternated between funny and disturbing and was thought-provoking.

Love, Stacey

To: Stacey D. Reynolds
Subject: Koby
Sunday, December 08

Hi, Stacey,

I had a dream you were here visiting and Koby came early. He was a chubby little guy, and he smiled at Grandma right away. I asked you, "How are you going to drive home? Do you have three car seats?"

I guess you talked to Laurie today. I talked to her later, and she said she couldn't believe no one told her that her sister was moving back to the Midwest.

Love, Mom

Subject: hi from Seattle
Thu, 12 Dec 2002

Hello,

Had a doctor's appointment on Tuesday and everything is going fine. I've gained about 20 lbs. so far. I am really starting to feel the extra weight, but I'm not overly tired.

Told my boss yesterday that I wasn't coming back after maternity leave. It just wasn't making sense for a lot of reasons. It is actually much cheaper for me not to continue working at this point. I told my sitter, too. She will work through January. I hope she can still come on occasion. The kids love her. I'm glad the kids are happy and adaptable. We will be putting them through a lot of changes in the upcoming months.

Stacey

12/23/02 6:28 PM

Hi, Mom and Gary,

Well, here I go. I was up at 6:00 am and went grocery shopping. Decided that was preferable to trying to do it with the kids later. For the rest of the day, I am determined to clean every last speck of mold out of my bathroom (probably a good thing to do whether I'm nesting or not!).

I have a difficult request for a last-minute present. Aleks is convinced his whale friend needs clothes. He is hoping Santa will bring some clothes for him. I am thinking of making some whale clothes out of some tiny baby T-shirts. Or should I just tell him he is silly and whales don't wear clothes?

Love, Stacey

Subject: doctor's appt.
Date: Tue, 7 Jan 2003

Hi, Mom

Just wanted to let you know my doctor's appointment went fine today. I am 1 cm dilated, and everything else is moving along. The doctor said the baby is sitting right on my bladder. No surprise to me. She said I could probably have the baby anytime, but she didn't think it would be for a couple of weeks. I am going to try to hold out till the 29th even though two weeks from now sounds awfully nice....

 I am alternating between really feeling on top of things and then feeling totally overwhelmed with everything that still needs to be done.

Had a great day with the kids. We painted this morning. Our kitchen is now an art gallery. Did you know that the easel can be used to make a nice little teepee when the painting is done? That kept the kids entertained for another half an hour.

Love, Stacey

Subject: allergies
Date: Fri, 24 Jan 2003

Hi, Mom and Gary,

I just called to get Kassia's allergy results. I know you were interested in hearing them. They just got them in. I guess the doctor hasn't reviewed them. The nurse said that it looked like eggs and wheat were still significantly high. Everything else seemed OK. I am really surprised about the wheat, but really, that has been the easiest to get around. The spelt flour works great. I'm relieved that the peanuts were low because that can be a very serious lifelong allergy. I've heard eggs can also be a quite serious allergy, but hopefully she will outgrow that. They are going to call after the doctor has had a chance to review the results. I don't think I'll go crazy and put cheese on her pizza tonight until we get the final word.

We are supposed to be in for a drenching weekend. The temp is supposed to remain in the 50's, though. I hope it stays warm for your stay. You will like it.

I've decided Sunday would be a good day for Koby to come if he decides to make an early arrival. We'll see.... I'll talk to you soon.

Stacey

Jakoby Allen Lesiewicz was born January 29, 2003. Grandma Carole arrived just in time that day from Wisconsin to help out as Stacey and Tommy were waiting and ready to head to the hospital.

Subject: hi from Seattle
Date: Mon, 17 Feb 2003

Hi, everyone,

Well, we are surviving. We sure do miss all our help, though. The kids got pretty sick over the weekend. Kassia has had fevers over 104 and Aleks has a bad cough and pink eyes again. I can only hope that breastfeeding will help the bug stay away from Koby. The doctor told me they routinely do spinal taps on infants under two months that have fevers over 100.4. I'm not going to worry about it too much. I took him to the doctor today because it looked like he might be getting pink eye. We don't know if that's what it is because it is very common for newborns to have goopy eyes. Anyway, the good news is he is growing like crazy. He already weighs over 10 lbs. and has grown 2 inches (can that be right?) in 2.5 weeks! He looks great, too. I'm waiting for the baby acne to start up—so far, so good.

Stacey

Sat, 1 Mar 2003

Hi, Mom,

I spent the afternoon taking the kids to the ice cream parlor and the park. We had a great time. The weather is so nice. Seattle is really taunting us.

As far as stopping in Boscobel, we will have to see what time of day we are coming through. It would be fun to make the stop. It would help convince Aleks we are moving closer to Grandpa and Grandma. Actually, we would be coming through north of there. We are doing our driving between 2 p.m. and midnight every day. We will also have to see how we are doing on days because we have to beat the moving truck, and then there is Tom's interview. He is anxious to get there and talk to the Harley guy. He sent his resume. The guy said he would just keep hiring until they were full. I guess we will have to stay in touch on our trip. After we have been on the road for 2–3 days, we will have a much better idea on how things are going.

We are doing a great job with packing, but I'm starting to freak about the cleaning now! I think if I line up some help with the kids, Tom and I can do it in two days.

Love Stacey

Subject: the packing continues
Date: Tue, 4 Mar 2003

Hi there,

Well we seem to be on track with our packing and everything, but we are getting to the point where every day/minute counts. Tomorrow our landlord is coming over. She wants to look around. She is also going to property manage our condo on a time and materials basis. Much cheaper than the $140 per month others charge, and she's good! The tenant will also sign another one-year lease—yeah!

Koby is sleeping. This seems to be the time of day when he takes a long nap (around noon). He is still gassy at night. I am experimenting to see if it is the beans or dairy (or neither). Heaven forbid it would be chocolate or the small amount of coffee I drink! Maybe he is just a gassy guy. He is doing well otherwise. I did get a couple of smiles, and he is starting to coo a little. Oh, my heart could just melt....

Aleks packed a couple of boxes in his room. He was a little better about seeing his toys go in boxes when he had some control.

I'm so excited. I've been trying to think of some way to work from home to generate a little extra income and have some fun, and something clicked this morning. I would like to design children's rooms and/or businesses that cater to children. I could rep some artists and products and make money selling their stuff, too. I could design a website and could do some of the work on line. It seems like a nice fit with my background in children's spaces and healthy interiors and my current work as a mom of three. I don't think I would want to have a store, but I guess that would be a possibility down the road. It would probably take me a year to get set up, but I'm excited about starting research right away.

Better go make use of my free hands.

Stacey

Stacey D. Reynolds wrote:

hello,

I'm getting excited about the move, but it is getting pretty crazy around here. the house is a mess and the kids are crabby, i think they're a little freaked too.

i found the coolest thing today. i have been really upset about leaving aleks' school, it has been a great experience for both of us. I found one just like it in elgin, that type of school is becoming a rarity in Illinois, so we are lucky. Apparently, we can still get in before the summer break in June then over the summer the families arrange play dates at parks so everyone stays connected. It would be a great way to meet people and make some quick friends for Aleks and Kassia.

Well koby is going into a bit of a collicky rage here. see if I can rock him back to sleep. I don't think he's pooped enough today.

Stacey (one-handed typing, baby on lap)

CHAPTER 11
Ho Jo's All the Way!

In 2003, because of a downturn in the tech industry and to be closer to family, the Reynolds/Lesiewicz family moved back to the Midwest. Tommy sold his Harley-Davidson motorcycle to help finance the move. They lived for a while in a house owned by Tommy's mother, Robin, in South Elgin, Illinois, and later purchased a home in Elgin. Tommy's first job in Illinois after the move was salesman at a Harley dealership.

Hi,

So far, so good. We have a few last-minute things to work out. Only one of them could potentially push our travel plans back. The car has to go in because the front blinker popped out. It seems they forgot a couple of screws when they did the body work. I hope they have the parts.

The kids and I are checking into a hotel this afternoon to take naps. Tom will be doing the final touches on the cleaning. We could probably have stayed here, but the carpets are a little damp.

If all goes well, we will be back here in the morning to check out. I have a doctor's appointment at 11:30, then we will hit the road after lunch. We will stay in touch.

Stacey

Sent: Monday, March 17, 2003
Subject: Re: travel update

Hi, Stacey and Tommy,

I guess if you read your e-mail before you take off tomorrow you will get this.

I'm picturing Stacey napping in the hotel with the kids while Tommy peels stickers off the fireplace.

Love, Mom

Subject: RE: travel update
Date: Tue, 18 Mar 2003

Hi, Mom,

Well, your vision was a little bit correct. The naps didn't happen. The kids were wired and were bouncing off the hotel room walls. They went to bed between 8:30 and 9. Tommy cleaned and entertained the neighbors who came over to get the futon and say their final goodbyes—yes, we gave that lovely thing (futon) away! He got to the hotel sometime between 11 and 12. I spent a lot of time peeling stickers off the fireplace last week, but I think I did it while gabbing on the phone.

It's 1 p.m. Tuesday. We are in the house still working on final cleaning touches and then have a few stops to make around town. We are toying with the idea of going as far as Spokane or Coeur d'Alene tonight and saving the big drive for tomorrow. I think that is wise if we don't get out of here until after 2. That will still put us in Billings tomorrow night. Gotta go.

Stacey

Subject: on the road
Date: Wed, 19 Mar 2003

Hi,

We are in Spokane. We left Seattle at 4:30 yesterday. We had to make a couple of stops to see that the cargo hold on top of the car was safe. It was loaded down and seemed a bit wobbly. We first went to the seller of the cargo holder. They said the cargo holder was fine but wanted to sell us some steel tracks instead of the factory tracks we have on the car. We then went to the car dealer and confirmed the factory tracks were doing just fine. So far, we haven't sent it sailing down the freeway, so I think it is just fine.

We rolled into Spokane at about 10 p.m. We were lured to a Howard Johnsons by a banner that said $39 rooms. We checked it out and found it was more like $69 for a family our size, but they had these great "kids Crayola" theme rooms with a VCR, an easel, crayons, fridge, microwave, internet, kid-size tables, and a free breakfast. It was perfect, and they take pets. We are now going to call and see if we can book Ho Jo's all the way down the line. They have these rooms in many of their hotels.

Look forward to seeing you.

Stacey

Subject: hi from South Elgin
Date: Fri, 28 Mar 2003

Hello,

Well, our place is looking a lot like a home.

We were just getting settled on Tuesday and felt like we had everything we needed and then on Wednesday all of our STUFF came. Oh, what fun to find places for everything. Actually, it is looking good.

We will be busy. The place is nice, but Jeff (Tom's brother) had a lot of projects in progress. In exchange for rent, we decided to do some work on the place and maybe replace some of the appliances (the oven isn't working). There will be some painting, we need to put railings on the exterior decks, there are some carpentry projects to finish, and we also want to do some gardening. The yard is huge!

Tom had his interview yesterday. He has a second interview with them on Monday. Their two top sales people are also from the computer industry. This dealership is ranked number 6 or 7 in the country for volume, and they are opening new stores. Tom was impressed with their business-like operation. There is room for advancement.... I hope the next interview goes well. He is excited.

We've done some exploring. I am really surprised at how much I like Elgin. South Elgin where we live was a tiny river community. There is not much to the original town except a town hall and an old train museum. They have train rides beginning in May. The town now has 16,000 people and is mostly subdivisions. There are three strip malls which have all of your basic services and a couple of good restaurants.

There is a bike trail one mile from our house that winds 61 miles through suburbs and forest preserves. I am anxious to try it out when I get my bicycle—if I get my bicycle. It was the only casualty of the move. They think it was misloaded with some items going to Detroit. If they find it, they are dropping it off on their way back through. The guys that drove the truck are the ones who loaded it in Seattle. We were very impressed with that company and glad we went with them and their fixed price. We would have been charged for an extra 1,300 lbs. if we had gone with Mayflower (but maybe I would have still had a bicycle!).

We drove into Elgin proper to take a look. It is not what I expected, which is good. Housing there is very affordable, and the place is loaded with lovely old Victorian houses. Most of them need some work. The downtown area is large and has nice old buildings, too. Many of the businesses were empty. It looks like everyone shops at Walmart and Target, a familiar problem, eh? They are building a large new library. They have a new symphony, a public museum, and a large new Parks and Recreation department that sounds like a cross between a fancy health club and a YMCA. It is evident some revitalization is taking place. Maybe a good time to buy???? The people seem racially diverse as well. Tommy and I both look at this as a positive.

You can take a train from Elgin to Union Station in downtown Chicago for under five bucks. That would be another plus.

I see the schools are a mess in this area due to budget cuts. They are cutting many "non-essential" programs. What a shame. This seems to be happening everywhere. They have an Einstein Academy here for gifted kids. I have no idea what it costs or what you have to put your kids through to get in, though.

We haven't heard from the preschool. I think they were on spring break this week. Hope we can get in to see next week.

All and all, I think we made a good move. Tommy seems to be happy, too. Of course, the best thing is being closer to you all. As soon as we get feeling a little more settled, we will plan a trip. We are wiped out—this has not been easy! I'll talk to you this weekend if we don't freeze to death. Brrrrrrrr, Stacey

Subject: grandkid report
Date: Wed, 9 Apr 2003

Hi, Mom and Gary,

Quite the news today. I'm glad the war will be over soon.

Koby went to the doctor today. He got so many shots; I feel sorry for him. He is very big—almost 15 lbs. and 26.5 inches. That puts him in nearly the 100th percentile in weight and height.

I got a swing after all. I think it will be the best $50 I ever spent.

Aleks and I went to his school today. I think I will really like the people. The kids seem to be good for the most part. Aleks typed his name on the typewriter. He wants to send it to you.

Aleks met more kids in the neighborhood. I'm just trying to decide how much running around I will let him do. He's gone out into the street a couple of times, which I don't like, and he wanders about four houses down to the other Alex's house. Alex seems like a pretty nice boy. I am completely cooked because he told Aleks that naps are for babies.

We've explored the area a little more. I went to a yoga class last night at the Rec Center. It is wonderful that you can drop in to any class for $5. It cost me $14 to take a yoga class in Seattle. I might try the butts and guts class sometime. I'm sure that would make me very sore.

Tom is out shopping for jeans. He starts work tomorrow. Exciting! His schedule is going to rotate on a monthly basis, I guess. Bike discounts are not part of the benefits package—only parts and accessories. The rest of the benefits are OK. Pay is fine if he sells a decent number of bikes, which we expect he will.

Stacey

Date: Tue, 29 Apr 2003

Hi, Mom and Gary,

This morning Aleks and I went on a nature walk for his school. The nature preserve down the road is a great place to take kids. They had plenty of interactive exhibits and a place for tired parents to sit and watch them. Since you have to walk down the trail to get to the center, it was not mobbed with people—we were the only ones there. On the path the guides pointed out the difference between regular dog poo and coyote poo (furry)—this was fascinating for the 3- and 4-year-olds.

Kassia went all day without a diaper yesterday. Tom has her dressed in overalls today. I think I'll go put some shorts on her.

I found some info on an artist's club like the one I was in in Milwaukee. I would like to do some work, maybe watercolor, to put in their fall show. It's non-juried, so anyone can be in it. They have meetings once a month. I also want to join a bicycle club that I found and go on some organized rides. It is hard to escape for the amount of the time it takes for a decent bike ride, though. We need to get some of those attachments and take the kids along. I think I will see if Lesley wants to do a big ride with me. There is one coming up at the end of June.

I better go. Aleks is having some kind of problem with his lunch. I also just missed the opportunity to change Kassia into those shorts.

Stacey

Subject: Happy Mother's Day
Date: Sun, 11 May 2003

Hi, Mom,

I'm glad we got to spend a little time with you before Mother's Day. Thanks for putting us up an extra night. It was nice to relax and visit with everyone.

We had a good ride home with just one stop. I think we have this driving with kids thing down. knock on wood. Stopping for food was pretty crazy. First, I pulled in and gassed up the car. Since it was a large and busy gas station, I had to unload the kids in order to go in and pay. Once inside, I ordered a sub for myself. The kids had their hearts set on Burger King across the street—that kind of fast food just doesn't sit well with me, so I was glad this place had sandwiches. While they were making the sandwiches, we went to the gas counter to pay for the gas. Aleks and Kassia asked for three different kinds of candy before we made it to the counter. After paying for the gas, I decided to make a break for the bathroom so off the four of us went. Of course, Aleks and Kassia had to go to the potty, too. After going myself, I assisted Kassia. I had to trust that Aleks was doing all right in the adjacent stall (such a big boy now!). Next it was time to wash all of our hands really good. The sinks were too high for the kids. Luckily, I had Koby in his car seat so I could hoist the other kids up to the sink and the soap. Once we were all clean, I went to retrieve my sandwich from the sandwich counter, and we were out of there. In the parking lot, there was an Army convoy. Aleks asked if they were "nice" Army guys. He decided for himself that they were because they didn't try to boom us. Now off to Burger King.

By this time, Koby is hungry and starting to cry. My plan was to go through the drive-thru, park in the parking lot, put the back hood up, and let Aleks and Kassia eat in the back of the car while I nursed Koby.

We went through the drive-thru. Unfortunately, their speakers weren't working well, and they could not hear me over Koby's cries which were getting very loud. They asked that I pull up to the cash window and place my order there. The car in front of us was taking too long, though. I could stand the cries no longer, so we maneuvered out of the drive-thru and pulled around to the front. We would have to go inside.

Koby calmed down a little while inside the restaurant. We ordered some kids' meals and then had to dispense our own drinks. I once again had to put Koby down on the floor to put the drinks together and then had to figure out how to carry the food, beverages, and baby seat and make sure Aleks and Kassia didn't get run over in the parking lot. I decided that the kids could carry their beverages while I carried the "happy meals" and Koby. I then set up the little picnic area in the back of the car for Aleks and Kassia. Koby is really wailing at this point while I fumble through the bags making sure Aleks got the plain burger with no mustard/pickles/and ketchup and Kassia's burger was extracted from the bun. I got more than a couple of stares. Once they were happily munching on their meals, I fed poor little Koby.

The rest of the way home was great. We laughed and sang, and I kept yelling, "Binkie, binkie!" to Aleks. As long as Koby had his plug, everyone was happy. Aleks did a super job of keeping it in.

We had to make an emergency pee stop for Aleks at Walmart just a few miles from home. You can pretty much repeat my second paragraph for this stop but add a temper tantrum by a 2-year-old in the middle of the parking lot. Yes, she was really laying herself down in the middle of the roadway. I got Kassia back under control by picking her up and pushing her in the shopping cart but did not get to the car without Aleks starting to cry (he wanted to ride in the cart, too) and Koby crying (pick the reason).

Once home, you think I would relax after such a day, but after hearing weather reports about the impending golf-ball size hail, I decided to empty the garage of something like 25 boxes so we could fit the car in it for the night. I worked like a little ant while Koby slept in the swing. I opened up a couple of boxes to reveal some of Aleks and Kassia's long lost treasures to keep them busy. I think Tommy thought I was crazy when he came home, but he went along with it. I told him I just raised our insurance deductible to $1,000 and was still feeling guilty about screwing up the checking account. The way our luck has been this week, it would really stink to have hail damage. If there was a way to save some cash, I would do it. Besides, it was great exercise.

As it turned out, we had only pea-size hail. We did have to hit the basement at about 11 p.m. when the tornado siren went off. That was exciting. Tommy was great. He was so calm with the kids. They did not even seem very frightened.

I better go. Koby woke up and is watching a Japanese children's program. He is not buying it. In fact, it is making him very angry. What if he starts speaking in Japanese?

Love and Happy Mother's Day from your daughter and one busy mom!

Stacey

Sent: Thursday, May 15, 2003

Hi, Mom and Gary,

The school is keeping me quite busy. I now hold three board positions for next year: secretary, forms, and equipment acquisition. There are a lot of people moving, so there is quite a bit of turn-over next year. I may be among the senior members the way it looks. I have the plans to work on the design for the new preschool space. I doubt there is any budget, though. The flooring really needs to be replaced, and with 1,900–3,000 square feet needed, that is no small job or price tag. I can see there are some fun things that could be done with paint in the rest of the space.

Stacey

Hello,

Tommy has plugged me in to a designer who is working with his company on their new design and image? I think she is a web designer. She has extended her services to help with the store front design and says they have architects working on the space but may need an interior designer. I have a lot of glitzy Harley stuff in my portfolio, which is now in their hands. We will see where it goes. If they want me to help, I will be in way over my head, but it will be fun! They are planning a move to a much larger location sometime this summer.

Tommy is selling lots of Harley's this week! He is really fired up. That is good because as I deposit his check today, we have $17 in our account (before the deposit). I think he has already sold enough to surpass our budget for next pay period, and he still has another week. Whew.

I'm working on starting my little business. I might e-mail my business plan to Gary and get his opinion and yours.

Today it is off to the bank, the grocery store, and the library. Robin has offered to come and sit for us tonight. There is a reggae band at the brew pub. It sounds like fun.

We looked at two duplexes this week. They were not large enough for us to live in. We will have to keep our eyes open and act on any large ones that come up. I've got a lot of information from co-op members on house hunting and neighborhoods. It seems everyone is buying and moving and is in about the same price range as us.

Kassia has now wilted on the floor and is crying. I think she needs some Mommy lap time, so I better move the laptop and let her sit on my lap instead.

Stacey

Sent: Saturday, May 31, 2003
Subject: hi mom and gary

Hello,

We had some weird weather last night. We were supposed to be in the clear and had no warnings, but the sky looked super weird. I went in and woke up the kids who were sound asleep at 8 p.m. just as the sirens started to go off. I freaked them out because I am not very relaxed about these things. Especially when I have a baby in my arms and two kids sleeping like rocks. I had to pull them by arms and more or less dragged them to the basement steps.

Tommy is off to work. There is a charity benefit. The Hooters girls are washing motorcycles for $10. Too bad it is 50 degrees, rainy, and very windy. They will probably be wearing sweat suits. Sorry, Tommy.

Stacey

Sent: Monday, June 02, 2003

Hi, Mom and Gary,

I got a lot done when Robin was here. I got the beginnings of a brochure written. It is hard to keep motivated. So far, I have a name, "Kid Scapes," the beginnings of a business card, an ad, and a simple business plan. I've done some research and have a list of stores in and around Chicago that I should visit. I've also bookmarked several websites. When we get our tax refund, I can get my cell phone, post office box, internet domain, printing and all that good stuff. I hope to get an ad in the August issue of *Chicago Parent*. I'm not sure I can be ready for business in late July, though, so maybe I'll wait a month.

Tommy was the #2 sales person this month. That is not bad going into his third month. I can't wait to get his check on Thursday. It is always such a mystery because we have no idea how much it is going to be until we get it. We just have to plan for the minimum although we know this one will be much more.

Koby found his feet and now grabs at them.

Kassia is back to diapers 100%. What am I going to do????

Aleks is playing garbage truck. He is always inspired by the garbage collectors on Monday mornings. Unfortunately, it means dumping as much as possible on the living room floor.

Stacey

Sent: Wednesday, June 25, 2003
Subject: he's moving

Mom and Gary,

Well Koby can scoot across the floor now... he does it on his back. I guess that would be a crab crawl or an upside-down seal. He also sits up for limited amounts of time.

I got this fancy cell phone for my business. With rebates, it was free. It takes pictures and video clips. Tommy is jealous of my new little toy.

Hot one today. We are watching movies and eating popcorn this afternoon in the air conditioning.

I'm on a waiting list for a natural-foods buying club. Sixty families meet at the American Legion in Elgin monthly to pick up their orders. We can buy at wholesale prices. What a nice little secret to find. I also found out about produce delivery like we had in Seattle. I am starting ours on the 6th. I'll have to start cooking again!

I better go. I have some preschool stuff to do. It looks like I will be donating services for the rest of the summer. It's fun and I'm meeting people.

Stacey

Sent: Saturday, August 02, 2003
Subject: hi

Hi, everyone,

We sure look forward to seeing you soon.

I have some good news and bad news. Tommy cannot make it on Wednesday. That is the bad news. The good news is that he is visiting the firm in downtown Chicago that he interviewed with last week. They want him to get the feel of what it would be like to work there for a day and get to know people. I think that is a pretty good sign. He thinks he will like it. He could commute by train from here. It's a recruiting job. He would be finding candidates for the many high-tech positions they have job orders for. That is what he is doing on Tuesday. On Wednesday, he is interviewing with a firm in Schaumburg. He has already had two phone interviews with them.

I'm really sorry. We will plan a trip to Wisconsin soon, and I will insist that we all go together! It is important he find a job now before the motorcycle biz slows down.

You are also all invited to come down for Koby's baptism on September 7. I don't expect it—it's a long drive for the day. I just wanted to let you know you are invited.

Koby had to see the doc today. His soft spot on his head was bulging after three days of high fever. That is a symptom of meningitis, so they wanted to check it out. We saw a nurse practitioner, two nurses, and two different docs during the visit. They decided he was too happy to have meningitis, but want him to come back tomorrow for another look. I think we are fine. His fever has subsided. I have decided the best cure for a child's fever is to take them in to the doctor for it. It usually goes away before you even reach the office.

Aleks and Kassia found some kiddy scissors and played beautician with each other's hair before Mom caught them in the act. Both have a few chunks whacked off the back. It looks really nice!

I've been painting clouds on the ceiling of the new preschool space.

I'll go now. I plan to make it to my exercise class tonight. I'm glad Koby looks and feels better so I won't feel guilty.

See you, Stacey

Sent: Thursday, August 07, 2003
Subject: hi

Hi, Mom and Gary,

I helped the woman next door put together party favors for her son's fourth birthday. She is due to have a baby any day and is planning a huge party for her son. There are three giant piñatas. There will be all kinds of Mexican food. I don't know how many are invited, but it is for adults and the kids. I put together 40 candy bags for the children. Poor woman is going to wear herself out! It is nice having Mexican neighbors. We have already been to one big party at another neighbor's for a high school graduation. They had Mexican beer and food and tequila shots (I passed on that one).

Happy birthday Gary!

Stacey (Gary and Stacey share an August 8th birthday.)

Sent: Saturday, August 09, 2003
Subject: hi

Hi, Mom and Gary,

Got my book and capris - thank you very much!

My birthday was fun. Tommy came home for lunch and brought me some frozen custard and made me an espresso. The kids and I went on a walk around the block and they picked me "yellow" and "white" things and gave them to me for my present.

The kids and Tommy are still next door at the party. I had to bring Koby home. It was bedtime. The food at the party was delicious. It was very spicy. They are breaking the piñatas now. I can hear them singing a song in Spanish every time someone tries to break it. Christine did not have her baby yet. Today is her due date. She was looking calm and happy. She must have worked her butt off to make all that food.

Stacey

Sent: Tuesday, August 12, 2003
Subject: new job

This is hot off the press. Tommy accepted the recruiting job in Chicago. He will start on Monday. Yippee! "My baby takes the morning train...."

Sent: Wednesday, August 20, 2003
Subject: hi from Stacey

Hello,

The preschool had a lively opening today. Kassia and Aleks got to meet some of the new kids who will be there. The school looked nice, even though some of the shelves need to be completed. The teacher's husband is also making a little house, which I will paint. It looks like we will have 14 or 15 students.

Koby is getting close to crawling. He is starting to push off with his legs but doesn't quite have the arm thing down yet. He is such a happy jolly little guy.

The kids are at such great ages. Never again will we have kids in these amazing developmental stages. It isn't easy at times, but it sure can be a joy at other times!

Kassia is so excited about going to the school. She is anxious to meet some "pink girls."

Stacey

CHAPTER 12

A 1928 Brick Bungalow

Sent: Sunday, September 28, 2003
Subject: house

Hi, Everyone,

We put in an offer on a house yesterday and today it was accepted. Whew! Now the excruciating financing and inspections. Wish us luck.... Our closing date is Nov. 7, just before the real cold sets in. At least we can have a leisurely move this time. I imagine we will be moving and unpacking right through the holidays.

The house is a brick bungalow built in 1928. Four bedrooms, 2.5 baths. The basement is partially finished. The lower level reminds me a little of our Milwaukee duplex. Wood floors, lots of wood molding, and a very similar layout. The upstairs has two bedrooms and a half bath. The garage is big (three car) and has a workshop and an attached sunroom. The yard isn't too big, but it does have some grapes, which will be fun. One thing that I like is that the house is a few blocks away from the preschool the kids are going to now and the elementary school Aleks will attend next year. It is also a reasonably short walk to the train station, so we may be able to get by with one car for a while.

We will keep you posted. I am sure it will be a busy month.

Stacey

Sent: Monday, November 10, 2003
Subject: the move

Hi, everyone,

Just a quick update. We spent the second night in our new home last night. It was a bit more comfy than the first night, since we were able to get our beds set up. I can't say we have slept well. I don't think I have had more than two hours of consecutive sleep in the past couple of nights. The kids have been sick (not bad, just cranky).

The house is absolutely wonderful. It seems so right for us. There is plenty of space. It was cool to settle in and watch the lunar eclipse and full moon the other night. The Jacuzzi tub has also been nice after the move.

We need to get some window treatments before the neighbors get to know us a little too well!

Love Stacey

Sent: Wednesday, December 24, 2003
Subject: Happy Christmas Eve!

Hi, Mom and Gary,

Whew, the kids were up at a little after 6 this morning. I can only imagine what tomorrow will be like. They are so excited.

It is amazing that the kids have not been bugging us about their Christmas wishes. It is actually really nice. Kassia mentioned once that she wanted a giant Barbie, and this morning she said she wanted Barbie everything, specifically Barbie pants, Barbie shirt, Barbie shoes. She did get a Barbie car. I could not resist it since it was a Volvo Cross Country just like ours. What a kick! It has car seats in it, so Barbie is going to have to get busy building her family soon.

I am not sure how we will peel these kids from their presents, but we plan on leaving at about 9 a.m. tomorrow. They may have a couple of things they can bring in the car to keep them busy.

See you tomorrow.

Stacey

Sent: Tuesday, January 06, 2004
Subject: must be sick

Grandma and Grandpa,

Aleks has been saying some really funny things since he has been sick.

At 1:30 the other morning, he woke up and was having a lively discussion with Daddy. One of the things he announced is that he knows how they take statues down. He said they tie a rope around it and pull on it. Daddy asked if he saw that on TV about Iraq. He said yes, "When they took the statue of that bad guy down."

About every hour, he comes up with something else he has been pondering in his feverish state.

Stacey

Sent: Thursday, January 08, 2004
Subject: the kids

The kids are doing better today. Koby had a little fever and was crabby so he went back to bed. I think he will be fine after more sleep. Later we will go outside and look at animal tracks in the snow. I think I saw some bunny and squirrel tracks. It will be good to get out of the house. I have seen so much Caillou and Arthur over the past couple of days my head could explode.

Stacey

Sent: Monday, January 12, 2004
Subject: well

Hello, Everyone,

What a week it has been! For the last week I have had at least one child if not all three running a temp of around or over 103. It started last week Sunday. Now eight days, 45 doses of Tylenol later, I think they are well.

Now I am ready to dig in and start painting and decorating the house. I think that the kids are already immune to every bug that is going around now. Hopefully they will stay healthy and can enjoy the rest of winter.

Love, Stacey

Sent: Sunday, February 15, 2004
Subject: Happy Valentine's Day

Hi, Mom and Gary,

Thank you for the Valentine's cards and money. The kids chose to spend their loot at the aquarium today. We had a WONDERFUL time. The kids were angels and there was a lot to see. Some highlights were seeing a scuba diver feed fish and swim with the manta rays, some big beluga whales, sharks and sawfish, and a live dolphin show. We spent about three hours and eluded a meltdown. Kassia crumpled at the front doors as we were leaving. Her newly purchased beluga "whale friend" fell on the floor as she was going through the revolving doors. Kassia thought it was fitting that she should also plant herself on the floor and refuse to get up.

I am recovering from an eye brow wax gone bad. I don't get them waxed often but have never had this occur before. Somehow, I got burned from the wax. I have red marks below my eyebrows, and it hurts. I'm even a little swollen. I want my money back.... My hair is red again also. I think I like it, but it is always scary to go out at first. It starts out very bright, but it fades quickly. It's good the aquarium was dark today, but I did hear some women say they liked my haircut. That boosted my confidence a little.

I got a call about a job. I handed out one business card at the preschool fair a couple of weeks ago and the woman called me. I have yet to touch base but hope we talk tomorrow.

Love, Stacey

Sent: Thursday, May 20, 2004

Hi, Mom and Gary,

Koby has learned the word "mine," complete with the gesture of pointing to his chest. The third one sure learns that word early.

I am watching Aliza now. Koby insists on having her sippy cup. His just will not do. We might venture out for a walk, but it is sure looking like rain.

I had a blast at the party last night. They served margaritas and had yummy food. I bought a pizza stone because we make pizza all the time from scratch. I would have been too confused if I started to pick out gadgets. There are so many. I was laughing when I came home because until a few years ago Tommy and I barely had measuring cups. We cook a lot, but we are in the dark ages as far as utensils, with the exception of our nice knife set. I met some more neighbors. They told me about their summer parties. We are really going to have fun.

I have a lot of work to do in the gardens if I am to continue Wende's, the previous owner's, legacy. The neighbors said she was out there all day every day. I am afraid I won't be able to keep up with that—I hope I don't let things go too much.

Now Aliza has Koby's cup. I guess they have traded. I think they need some attention now. I better go.

Love, Stacey

Sent: Tuesday, May 25, 2004
Subject: hello

Hi, Mom and Gary,

Aleks asked me what I want to be when I grow up. He wondered if I wanted to be a gas station worker. He said he wants to be a gas station worker or a teacher because they are both safe things. After thinking about it a minute, he changed his mind. He said that gasoline is flammable, so a gas station person would be dangerous. I guess we settled on a teacher.

I completed the worst part of my project upstairs today while all three kids took a nap. About 30% of the ceiling in the office/soon-to-be guest room upstairs needed to be scraped. It was a time-consuming and messy task. Now I have to patch it, prime it, and paint it with textured paint. It will be quite a transformation when it is done. There are still some coins super-glued to the ceiling. I have to figure out how to get those down. I told Aleks I hope he never does that.

Stacey

Sent: Friday, June 11, 2004
Subject: hi

Hi, Mom and Gary, how are you?

Little Koby is sure changing. I can't wait until you see him. His skin is getting brown (bad mommy for not putting enough sunscreen on), and his hair is blonder. He is getting a full mouth of teeth, and he has little curls that I refuse to cut. He likes to climb on top of things and yell as loud as he can. He also likes to dance.

Kassia inherited a Little Tikes kitchen from the neighbors across the street. It is huge, but I think it is something she will get a lot of enjoyment out of.

Aleks has been busy creating. This morning he made paper clothes for his whale friend, a Barbie paper doll for me, several Father's Day drawings including a picture of Daddy on a motorcycle, and out of Legos he made a fancy ice cream truck that goes in the water and flies and squirts chocolate out of its back end. Yum.

Love, Stacey

Sent: Saturday, June 26, 2004
Subject: dancing

Hi, Mom and Gary,

Kassia had her first dance class today. My eyes welled up when I saw her out there. She did such a good job and wasn't afraid. I could tell she was trying to do her very best. They were asked to do a crab crawl across the room. She went all the way across the room and back. I think she was the only one who completed the task. She also did an excellent little twirl. It's early to say, but we might have ourselves a little dancer.

Aleks started another round of Kyuki-do. He is doing great, too. He had tee-ball on Monday night. The instructor is excellent. I think it is a much better class than he was in last summer.

Tommy and I are going to a movie tonight. We plan on seeing Fahrenheit 9/11. A little bit of liberal propaganda to taint our minds. I always find Michael Moore's movies/documentaries entertaining. I can't wait.

Stacey

Sent: Wednesday, August 25, 2004
Subject: school day

Hi, Mom and Gary,

It is 6 a.m. and guess who is up getting ready for school today, Mommy? I think I have butterflies in my stomach. Aleks is still sound asleep. The kids slept through the night. I did not think they would as we had stormy weather last night. Between 6 and 7, the tornado sirens went off three different times. We would go to the basement and then come up, and I would say, "See, it's all over," and then 20 minutes later, they would go off again. Poor Aleks looked very traumatized.

Oops, sounds like someone is awake. I am going to get started with breakfast. My kitchen still needs picking up from last night. I have to make sure we give Aleks the proper send-off this morning.

I will probably call or e-mail with a full kindergarten report later.

Stacey

Aleks' First Day of Kindergarten

I wake up this morning at 5:50 and bound out of bed. It is Aleks' first day of school, and I have much to prepare. It is another 30 minutes before my kindergartener crawls out of bed. I greet him exuberantly at his bedroom door. His response is: "Stop staring at me Mom." By 7, I have made Tom and myself our morning coffee, waffles are in the toaster, and Aleks has started getting dressed.

Things start taking a twist at around 7 a.m. just as Tom leaves for work. First, I make a last-minute decision to wash the little T-shirt that Aleks needs with his school supplies. It becomes clear it is going to be nowhere near ready by 8:15. It is amazing how long it can take one little shirt to dry in the dryer.

I start getting the kids dressed one by one. First is Aleks. He is ready and standing by the door by 7:45. He looks fabulous. He combed his own hair and asked for a washcloth to wash his own face. What a big boy! Next is Kassia. She insists on wearing her school dress, too. We find that it is in the wash. She is cooperative and lets me pick out an outfit for her. She is dressed and ready to go. It is 7:50 now. I check the dryer one more time. Aleks' shirt is still not dry. I take a peek at myself in the mirror. I am not dressed, and I haven't showered. I decide that my new short hair will pass for really curly this morning.

A last-minute double check of the school supplies reveals a small problem. While playing with his backpack and messing around with his supplies, Aleks packed his Elmer's glue with the lid open. Everything in his backpack is stuck together. I am surprised Aleks takes this in stride. I tell him we will tell the teacher and bring some different supplies tomorrow. Actually, we are able to separate all of them and peel the glue off with the exception of two pencils, which are hopelessly glued together.

It is 8:00. I turn my attention to Koby, who needs his diaper changed and needs to get dressed. He has a big poopy diaper that requires more than a little bit of cleaning. This sets me back a little, but soon he is dressed and ready to go. It is 8:10. I look at myself in the mirror again and decide my hair will not pass as pleasant and curly. Instead it has that distinct just crawled out of bed look. So, it will be. I need to get dressed. We need to leave in five minutes. My jeans are in the wash, so I put on a pair of dress slacks and my clogs. If I look like I am dressed up, maybe people won't notice my hair.

We make it out the door at exactly 8:15. Aleks has already seen a couple of his friends go past our house. Koby and Kassia hop in the wagon while the big boy walks. We arrive at the school at 8:25. The teacher is outside greeting students and parents. I get caught up in conversation with a couple of parents and never get to meet the teacher. She looks nice, though. Aleks and the other kids look happy and eagerly wait in line with their oversized backpacks hanging off them. The bell rings, and the teachers take the children into the school. I notice a few more tears on the parents' side than the kids. I have a couple little tears myself. They look so big and independent marching into the school. Once they are inside, I realize I have forgotten a bag with a couple of Aleks' supplies. I get into the school just before they lock the doors and deliver the goods to his classroom. At least I get a good peek at the room. The teacher has already begun her introduction. Aleks does not notice his weird, messy-haired mom in the back delivering the forgotten items.

Kassia, Koby, and I pack up in the wagon. The faint sound of thunder rolls overhead as we start our trek home. Kassia wants to play when we get home and relishes the attention she is getting. She announces that she wants to be a teenager or maybe just five years old. I ask her if she wants to go to school like the big kids and she says, "Yes." Koby colors with us and consumes half a rainbow crayon before we have to pack up at 10:45 and make the trip again.

There are sprinkles in the air that we aren't prepared for. Fortunately, the real rain holds off for us. The teachers bring the children outside at 11 a.m. and they are told they can go when they see their parents. Aleks has a big smile on his face. I try to do a little interview with the video camera. When asked how his first day was, he simply says "Good." When asked what they did, he says, "We just talked." He looks happy—that is what is important. I'm not able to capture the moment with the video camera as I would have liked because in one arm is the camera and with the other arm I am trying to restrain Koby who is threatening to escape onto the playground. I also ruin the video by accidently hitting a button on the camera. Aleks' first day of school will be labeled inappropriately as "happy birthday."

Aleks is tired and wants to ride in the wagon on the way home. I guess his first day wiped him out. We are about halfway home and heading downhill when I trip on the sidewalk. Those darn clogs! I do everything I can to keep from falling down and crashing onto the video camera. Fortunately, I recover a couple of feet from the ground. I have lost my grip on the wagon which continues to career downhill until I stop it with my leg. The whole thing stops with a jolt. Kassia and Koby are pretty shook up. Kassia bumps her arm a little, but it isn't long before we all look at each other and laugh.

An eventful morning it was. I better get used to this. We have about 180 more mornings to go. I developed my own little report card for the day.

Uses time wisely: D-
Appearance: D+
Overall preparedness: F
Kids' appearance: A
Kids are happy: A

Sent: Tuesday, September 14, 2004
Subject: hi from Stacey

Hi, Mom and Gary,

I got a weird call today. The Environmental Home Center burned down last month. It was pretty much a total loss. They are rebuilding the business and want some help with their showroom design. I said I would help. I'll work out some kind of trade for compensation. It was good to hear from him again. He was pretty upbeat given the circumstances.

School's going well. Aleks says his favorite part is recess—typical boy. He told me he spends his recess in an unusual way, though, under the play unit with Emma telling secrets. He told me that he can't tell me the secrets. The only one he can tell is that he and Emma are friends. If Emma's father wasn't a minister and her mother a social worker, I might be worried....

I locked me and the kids out today. I had lots of offers to help me get in but found I was able to break into the kids' bedroom in less than two minutes. No tools, just a ladder. That is re-assuring, isn't it?

Stacey

Sent: Tuesday, October 26, 2004
Subject: candy snatchers

Candy has been disappearing faster in our house than explosive stashes in Iraq. Two days ago, Tommy found a stash of candy in Aleks' secret drawer that looked suspiciously like our Halloween candy. We busted him! I left the bag down within reach, and the little stinker got into it while I was out raking leaves.

Today it was chocolate chips. I could tell something was up by how whispery Aleks and Kassia were. I went to the window sill where they were huddling and found a pile of chocolate chips. When confronted, they lied to me. We then talked about the story of Pinocchio.

At least I can say that our little pirate and Barbie princess (and little Batman) are ready for Halloween. It should be fun, and I think everyone will have their fill of candy by the end of the week.

Stacey

Sent: Tuesday, March 9, 2005
Subject: all in a day

Hi, Mom and Gary,

Well my afternoon watching five kids did not end without an exciting visit by the Elgin Police Department. One of the children (no one is 'fessing up) dialed 911 during some innocent pretend play involving police. After probing the room for evidence, I saw sheets of paper where both Kassia and Grace had scribed their names and 911. Apparently, the culprit knew what they were doing.

The suspects were lined up for some sofa time. I retreated to the kitchen and had a couple spoonful's of Ben & Jerry's ice cream. I don't know if it looked more like a scene out of *Desperate Housewives* or

Super Nanny. I went for a walk tonight, and it definitely had the neighbors asking questions.

Stacey

Sent: Thursday, March 11, 2005
Subject: hi

Hi, Mom and Gary,

Mom, I forgot to tell you about the art portfolio Aleks brought home the other day. I had been asking him what he does in art because he hadn't brought anything home. Yesterday he came home with a whole portfolio of beautiful projects. They were all really nice! I will save them, so you can see. Most were mixed media. They were planned projects, but it looks like there was room for plenty of creativity. I was a little baffled by his "self-portrait." I did not know what to say. His portrait looked like a picture of an African American girl. Either he doesn't have his grandmother's talent for portraits, or he was sitting across from his friend Emma—it looks a little bit like her.

Stacey

Sent: Wednesday, April 13, 2005
Subject: Re: Hello

Hi, Mom,

It has been a busy time lately. Where do I begin? For one thing, the weather is nice, and we have been out in the yard a lot. I am finding I can get more done this year with the kids outside.

Saturday, Kassia started another gymnastics series and then we went to a birthday party. It was a miniature golf party for one of Aleks' friends. Kassia and Koby and I hung out in the mall while it was happening. We were all pretty tired by the end of the day.

Sunday, I went to the Unitarian church. I am doing a little intro class there and so far, really like it. It is amazing the diverse backgrounds and belief systems that people come from. Later we celebrated

Grandma Robin's birthday at Jeff's house. We had perogies and a Dairy Queen ice cream cake.

Aleks and I are now in a family Kyuki-do class. It is fun for us to go together, and I like the feel of getting back into martial arts. I hope to push him along a little so that he can earn a belt soon.

Tonight, is Aleks' first soccer practice. I went and got all the gear last night. This is a sport that I am not very familiar with. He is convinced that he wants to do it. It will be fun but busy for the next six weeks. There are a lot of games and practices. I guess I am now what they call a soccer mom.

We made some progress on the floors upstairs over the weekend. I imagine the sanding will finally be done this weekend, so we can finish it next week. I did another little painting for Kassia's room. Slowly we are getting some things accomplished.

Stacey

Sent: Friday, May 13, 2005
Subject: hi

Hi, Mom,

I am picking out an outfit for Kassia to wear to a little birthday party tonight. That can be tricky. She wants to wear her sweater all the time now. Even though it has been a little cooler the last couple days, I don't think it is sweater weather. Hard to tell a four-year-old that. We are going over to the neighbors to celebrate their daughter's sixth birthday.

Tomorrow Kassia will go to her big party. They are going to a little studio and having their hair, nails, and age-appropriate make-up done and then dress up for a fashion show. My little girl might never be the same after all of that! I hope I can get pictures.

We have a full day on tap tomorrow. We have gymnastics in the morning, then Aleks has a birthday party to go to in the afternoon. We are also having a bake sale/car wash for the preschool. I am hoping Tom can mow the lawn at the house in South Elgin and make some headway on sanding the hallway upstairs, but I will not dictate what he does with his spare time. Oh, maybe I will hint around a bit....

Sunday promises to be a little calmer. I have to go to church because they have a new member welcoming party. I joined the UU church. I've met a lot of really nice people there who have similar values. We will still go to the Catholic church occasionally. The kids will do religious education at both places. They will have their Christian foundation but will learn about other belief systems, too. Godparents need not be alarmed! I'm happy—I think it completes the puzzle of our move two years ago.

Love, Stacey

Sent: Thursday, June 02, 2005
Subject: hello

Hi, Mom and Gary,

On Tuesday night in a rush to go to kickboxing, I backed into Tommy's car. I think he has had it home and all repaired for four days and now it has another nice dent. It will cost us at least another $1,000 as that is our deductible. I don't know if we will run it through insurance or not.

The good thing is that the Volvo lived up to its reputation (built like a tank) and only sustained some bumper scratches.

Tommy may switch from his HR/IT/recruiting position to sales. Business has been slow at their company, so they are not doing any new recruiting and need him more in sales. It will be more stressful for him. I know he will do well, though.

I planted some more red impatiens in the corner by our kitchen today. I think that is our wealth area of the house for feng shui. I wonder where the sleeping area is?

Stacey

Carole: During a visit to a neighborhood antique store Stacey discovered and later purchased an intriguing urn, which she believed was Moroccan and worth more than the marked price. Her interest in Moroccan décor was inspired by a trip she and Tommy took in 1998.

Sent: Thursday, July 21, 2005
Subject: hi

Hi, Mom,

The kids have been parading around the neighborhood this week. On Tuesday, they all marched down the sidewalk in costume looking for trick or treat candy (clever, aren't they?). Yesterday all of the neighbor kids attended a birthday party for Gus Gus, a guinea pig who celebrated his second birthday.

I've had some interesting "finds" this week. One was at the antique store. The other was in our backyard. I checked out a new antique store in the neighborhood on Tuesday with all three kids in tow. I found an intriguing urn and had a strong hunch that it was from Morocco. I asked the shop owner if it was from Morocco or Mexico. He had no idea, but a woman who was pretending to be an expert concluded that it was from the Southwest U.S. and was an American Indian piece. It was priced at $75. I went online and found Moroccan antiques that looked very similar. The prices ranged anywhere from $600-$1,600. It was glazed with polychromatic glazes and had silver and leather accents. I might see if they will take $50 for it and call it my birthday present.

The other find was a hummingbird moth in our backyard. The kids and I were in the backyard at dusk admiring some pink clouds remaining after sunset. Over on the phlox, there was what appeared to be a hummingbird. After a closer look we determined it was an insect. A Google search verified that it was a clearwing hummingbird moth. It was really cool. It was almost magical because the kids and I stood right by it and analyzed it. The sky and the flowers were so pretty, too. I guess they aren't uncommon. I don't think I have ever seen one though. Have you?

Tom works until 10 tonight. I am glad it is cool so I can throw a pizza in for dinner. The kids will be very happy with that, and I won't have to make a big dinner. I'm trying to get Koby to sleep. It will be a long evening if he is crabby and decides to be a mean Batman—or as he would say Batbam.

I'll talk to you soon.

Stacey

Morocco, 1998

Following are some excerpts from Stacey's Moroccan story written after the 1998 trip.

February 11

We landed in Casablanca at 7:30 a.m. local time after a relatively short 6 hour and 20-minute flight from JFK. The sun was just beginning to rise over the rain-soaked plains. As our 747 jumbo jet swooped down for a nearly perfect landing, I caught glimpses of homes and farmhouses in a style I will become very familiar with over the next week. Most of the structures were stone and stucco designed around a central courtyard. The austere white edifices of these buildings contrasted sharply with the rich green landscape. This is not how I pictured Morocco.

From our arrival at the gate, we were ushered into a transit lounge to obtain boarding passes for our next flight. Thus far, we've been able to get by speaking only English. This is good because after two nights of flying as well as twelve hours of wandering around Manhattan, I'm lucky if I'm awake enough to speak my own native tongue. A look around the airport tells me we have lost most of the American tourists who were on our earlier flight. I think most hopped on a connecting flight to Tunisia. For some reason, this pleases me. I picked up an issue of the local newspaper, *Le Matin*, that was left on an adjacent seat. I scanned the headlines, which included three stories about the tensions in the Gulf but fortunately nothing about Monica Lewinsky. At least that is behind us! I could decipher the French in the articles enough to understand the gist of the articles on the Gulf but could not pick up on any of the "tone" that the articles were written in. Within minutes, we boarded our connecting flight to Agadir.

The flight to Agadir took us over more farmlands. I could see the Atlas Mountains in the distance. Gradually the landscape became more arid but still less desert-like than I had imagined. Our flight landed at a modern well-kept airport in Agadir. We landed in what I thought looked like a parking lot. Our plane was emptied, and we walked through two giant front doors flanked by security police.

The lines in the airport ran efficiently although we were the last passengers to pass through the customs official. I responded nervously when he asked me "Chicago?" I was confused and said, "No, Madison, Wisconsin." He had read on Tommy's entry information that he was born in Chicago and merely wanted to tell us he had a friend that lived there. We smiled and proceeded to get our luggage.

Our luggage came through the carrier promptly. I have been super impressed with Royal Air Maroc and this airport. The service so far has exceeded that of most U.S. airlines I have been on. A tired-looking American couple with an infant child walked in front of us as we approached a man with a fez and white robe holding onto a "Vultar" sign (our hotel). Later we will befriend these people, but for now our conversation is limited to small talk. I am too tired and awestruck with my surroundings to communicate right now. On the way to the hotel, we see men and women dressed in their traditional garb. Donkeys, sheep, and even a few camels are along the roadside. The architecture appears Spartan on the outside with walls, walls, and more walls. The sun is shining, and the colors are more beautiful than I ever imagined, reminding me a little bit of the more arid parts of Oahu in Hawaii.

After about 20 to 30 minutes of driving we arrive at Club Vultar, our hotel. Like the brochure, it was grand and beautiful—a lush oasis in contrast to the poverty and confusion on the outside. We are a little confused at first. Everyone here speaks Italian. The French phrases I practiced were useless in this resort. Anyway, we managed to get our room key. After showering, we walked around the club to orient ourselves. At this point, I felt as if I was a zombie walking among a mix of energetic and attractive young Italian staff and middle-aged European sun worshippers. One staff member mentioned that there aren't too many Americans staying here right now, but on Saturday, 45 more will arrive. I got the impression the club is pressing hard to open up the American market and the feeling they are going out of their way to accommodate. We feel very welcome.

• • •

February 12, Marrakech

Our wake-up call this morning was at 5:00 a.m., well before sunrise. It seemed unnatural to be waking at this hour, but the anticipation of the day ahead was enough to keep us going. Just before we left the room, I heard some strange chanting emerging through the balcony doors. Though the chanting seemed very powerful, it was tinny as if it was being projected over a microphone, I quickly dismissed it and we were off to our bus.

The bus pulled away from the hotel at 6:00 sharp. A long introduction was first given in Italian, German, and finally English. Of the 25 people on the bus, almost all were Italian. There were a handful of Germans and we were the token English-speaking Americans. Our Moroccan guide Kareem spoke English and three other languages very well. I felt both guilty and blessed with the fact that he went out of his way to make sure we understood everything. He explained that our trip would take us over the Anti Atlas Mountains and then down to a plain. The city of Marrakech is considered one gateway to the Sahara. The trip will take approximately three hours. We will spend a full day in Marrakech and return around midnight.

• • •

Half a roll of film later, we arrive at El Bahia Palace. I am even more amazed at the level of architectural detail. This palace was built in the late 19th century by a couple of sultans. All of the ceilings were cedar painted in intricate symbols using only natural pigments for the paints. Large cedar doors were intricately carved. Aside from these features, the story behind this palace was interesting. Inside were a series of secret chambers for the sultan and all of his concubines. The large inner courtyard was "the courtyard of the 24 concubines," although I counted 30 doors surrounding us. I wondered what the other six doors were for. Nonetheless, this was a very busy man! Kareem briefed us on polygamy and their culture. I respectfully acknowledged this without comment and wondered if he noticed my slight embarrassment. Polygamy is actually somewhat rare today since you must gain the approval of your other wives before you bring another on board. I wonder what could possibly convince a woman to allow this. He also expressed in jest that most men today feel one wife is plenty!

We wander into another even more beautiful courtyard reserved for the sultan's four favorite concubines and his wives. There was room for favoritism.

• • •

The next few hours were my most memorable in Marrakech and perhaps on the whole trip. As we filed off the bus, this was yet another time our group had no idea what awaited us. As we passed under the fortified gate and into the medina, the sunlight gave way to semi-darkness. We were immediately accosted by a number of children and other well-wishers who offered their services. One small girl approached me and managed to divert my attention by pointing to her henna tattoo. This allowed her enough time to tie a piece of braided lace around my arm. She insisted it was a present but would not leave until we gave her a dirham (10 cents). It was slightly annoying at the time, but now I look at it as a small price to pay for this scraggly piece of lace which is now a tangible memory of that day. As our group was swallowed up by our strange surroundings, we noticed that our "snake" had doubled up and many of the couples in the group were now holding hands. I believe it was less romance than fear of the unknown that caused this phenomenon.

The sights, smells, and sounds that swept over us could not be duplicated in any setting. Not only were goods being sold, but goods of all types were being manufactured all around us. Your eye could wander down a corridor and see beautiful wool yarns drying in the sunlight. Next you may be surrounded by metal workers and metal objects of all types. Giant star-shaped mosque lamps hang above while sconces, chairs, and candle holders lie below. The crazy rhythmic clanking of the metal workers, the general filth of these metal working men, and the smoke from the occasional welder is a scene I won't soon forget. I will never look at those inexpensive metal objects found at stores like Pier One and Cost Plus without thinking of this place. At one point, we saw a hip-looking Caucasian woman and her equally hip-looking male counterpart seated on the ground with one of the workers. They were showing the gentlemen their book of chair designs and other art objects. I imagined them negotiating a contract to make chairs for their gallery in Soho, chairs that here they could purchase for a few bucks and maybe sell for over $100 in the U.S.

My only regret about this strange tour is that we had to keep pace with our group. At one point, I backtracked a few steps for a Kodak moment but was quickly prompted back into the tour by our guides. They knew that to lose someone in this maze would be a disaster.

· · ·

We rejoined our group and were informed that we will now go to Place Djemaa el Fna. This is a giant square in the middle of Marrakech that I have read and heard about so much. It's difficult to tell what time of day it is walking down the narrow dark street of the medina, but I am excited thinking we will be there at sunset when all the magic begins.

And magic it was. The square was full of people, and the last rays of sunlight were bouncing off the Cafe Le France. As I looked around, the first thing that struck me were the number of maimed people. A row of blind men sat in front of us, a sick child begged for money. I pitied them but stayed well away! Groups of people surrounded magicians, soothsayers, tumblers, and snake charmers. Drum beats and tambourines gave the square a pulse. The sun gradually sunk below the horizon as smoke from food stands of searing flesh of all kinds filled the air. We walked past the booths where hanging carcasses were on display. I tried to figure out what each of the meats were but could not always identify. Some medium-shaped heads were lined up that looked like cats or dogs; more likely, they were lamb. It's hard to tell when they don't have ears. Men, women, and children sat around the booths and consumed the meat not unlike a hot dog stand at a county fair. We were to rejoin the group at 6:30 for dinner, but I doubted we would be eating here. We enjoyed a view of the square from the balcony of Cafe Glacier. It was dusk now and once again I heard chanting. The mosque was located across the street, and the muezzin was calling all Muslims for the required fourth (of five) prayers of the day. The faithful headed to the mosque in droves as the chants were broadcast through yet another tinny microphone. Not long after that, a full moon rose over the square in the East right over the mosque. All things said, this was a really cool experience.

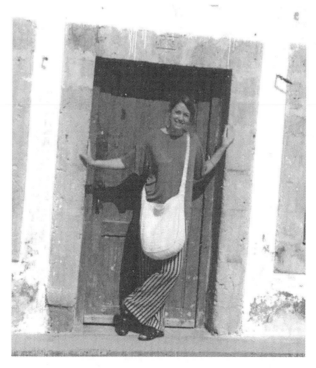

• • •

Next, we were approached by a nicely dressed gentlemen who asked to be our guide for the price of some cigarettes or a small meal. We explained that we wanted to look around by ourselves. He was pleasant and not pushy. He smiled and left us alone. After a soda and a brief discussion in another open air, fly-ridden establishment, we decided to hire this man as our guide. It would be a quick and efficient way to hit the main spots of this town and a sure way to get roped into buying something. After introducing ourselves to our trusted guide, Abdul, we let him lead the way to the market. I looked back nervously as several men in a nearby doorway yelled "Soud, soud!" (rhymes with could) I had no idea what that meant, but it seemed to be directed towards us. Was it some sort of warning? I decided we were safe with this guy as long as we stayed out of back alleys. Abdul's English was adequate. We asked a few questions back and forth, but he didn't explain anything of historical significance. I think back to my guide book and remember that this is the city of the women who wear blue. Sure enough, they were there in beautiful indigo veils, contrasting nicely with the pink buildings. It is also called "Little Marrakech" and is known for its slightly more laid-back version of Marrakech souks. Supposedly the tourists are not as exploited here. Well....

After about ten minutes of meandering through endless stalls, we were greeted by a man who went out of his way to lead us into his shop. For the first time, Abdul encouraged us to stop and look around. This was probably "his" shop. He would get a commission on anything that we purchased. Some bracelets caught my eye immediately, and some serious bargaining ensued. Once we settled on price, the salesperson wrapped them and then beckoned us back to the adjoining rug gallery. Up until this point, we had avoided these rug galleries. However, these salespeople had won our trust. We wandered back slowly, both knowing we would not walk out without a rug. I secretly wanted a small rug and had a set price in my mind on what I would spend. It was interesting to observe how their sales tactics unfolded as dozens of kilims were unfolded in front of us. I held back any expression of interest but as soon as

Tom reached to touch one of the rugs, the salesperson asked Abdul to get us some mint tea. He knew he had us! Next the salesperson brought us the guest book and explained that the U.S. singer Sade was a repeat customer of his. Inside the tattered guestbook was a photo of the singer with Abdul. If Sade shopped here, of course we must! I wondered why he did not have us sign his guestbook.

Amazingly, after going through a process of elimination, Tom and I agreed that we liked the same rug. Everything was moving along as if choreographed. Next came the awkward bargaining. As in all of our transactions, the dealer started with a ridiculously high price. I shyly responded with a much, much, lower price, which was a little under what I wanted to pay. I was pleased when we settled on a price that was only slightly higher than the number in my mind, if you didn't include the commission of 200 dirhams ($20 U.S.). This commission is for the shop-keepers who made this great deal possible for us while all the profits go to the rich owner who was only present in a gold-framed portrait hung precariously over the cash register. I've read these commissions are typical. It is all part of the deal. We paid with our Visa. We will know in about a month whether or not this was a huge mistake. Tom made sure to get a business card with the shop name and phone number, which we kept safely with the credit card receipt. All in all, this was a fun experience, once we let go of our inhibitions and allowed ourselves to be swept up under the spell of the magic carpets. Nonetheless, we rationalized the purchase all the way back to the car thinking at the very worst our purchase would have cost the same in the U.S., but the experience would never be the same! We will always remember the taste of that mint tea and the smell of those musty rugs in that gallery.

• • •

Tonight, as we've done for the last five nights, we went across the street for a beer before dinner. Abdulah and company were working again. There was something about us that amused them. Like the other nights, we caught them staring at us and whispering to each other in their language, occasionally chuckling. Was it something about the way we looked? Did they think it was peculiar how we came there every night at the same time and unlike the other tourists, we sat up at the bar? Did one of them have a crush on me? I guess we will never know. We explained to Abdulah that this was our last night. He announced this to the others. "American," he said. They all waved, and I held back a tear as we headed back to the hotel.

. . .

February 18

We woke up surprisingly early. Both of us called in to work opting to take the day off. We need to find our luggage and get situated before attempting to connect with the real world again. We take this unique opportunity to have lunch together at one of our favorite neighborhood spots, Mamas Mexican Cantina. The cheese-laden food here is heavy compared to what we have been eating this week, but as always it goes down very well when accompanied by a Corona. We sat back and reminisced. Our long flight makes Morocco seem very, very, far away from us now.

Should the sound of the tambourines or the echoes of the muezzin ever fade from our memory, we will always have the Moroccan CD's that we purchased at the record store. We returned home to find our luggage had been delivered. We opened one of the CD's and played it as I unwrapped the rug which was safely tucked in one of my suitcases. The musty smell of the rug gallery in Taroudant filled our living room as we admired the rug's intricate weave.

There is no doubt Morocco will always be in our hearts as well as on our living room wall. I would like to return some day. First, I would study French to enable myself to connect with the people of Morocco on a more intimate level. At the same time, I feel the need to travel to other parts of the world knowing there are probably many places equally as fascinating and as easy on the pocket book! For the next year, I will be content in my own backyard exploring the beauty of the Northwest and also returning to my familiar surroundings in the Midwest, the place I really consider home.

CHAPTER 13
Costa Rica, 2005

Sent: Wednesday, July 27, 2005
Subject: birthday

Hi, Mom,

For birthday ideas, I put three books on my Amazon wish list—two are on natural houses and one is on gardening. I can't think of much else. I always need clothes. I will definitely need a coat this fall. I would also love to go in for a massage some time. There is a place in Elgin called Simple Balance Holistic Center. Maybe a gift certificate from there towards a massage.

Had tree trimmers here on Monday. We were leaving for swim lessons as the limbs started dropping. I was so worried about what the men were doing that, in a hurry for our first lesson, I backed out of the garage with the hatch open on the car. It hit the garage door. (Remember, Tom spent the whole weekend installing the new opener.) Fortunately, the damage to the garage door was minimal, and the opener still worked. The car is kind of OK. The hatch opens but catches in the middle. There is a dent across the hood of the car, but it is a straight line and it looks like it was supposed to be there—Tom says, "until the paint starts peeling on it at least."

Needless to say, it was a disturbing day all around. It was a shock to see how many nice live limbs they cut, but once the debris was clear, I calmed down about it. There are a couple of sunny openings that will probably benefit my garden. I just love those trees, though.

Love Stacey

To: Carole Young
Sent: Monday, August 08, 2005

I really like the idea of not having a car this week and just hanging out with the kids and doing gardening and stuff, but I felt a little stranded on my birthday.

The kids made me all kinds of little pictures and gave me necklaces and Tootsie Rolls. Tommy sent me a dozen roses (what a stinker). We had our pizza party and a little dance party tonight. It really was not a bad day. I am very lucky.

I like the idea of being 41. I feel like now I am "in" my forties. I don't mind getting older. I see how much wiser and creative you have become. I look forward to that!

Love Stacey

Sent: Wednesday, August 24, 2005
Subject: first day

Hello, Everyone,

Aleks had his first day of school and things went without a hitch. No spilled glue or problems of any sort.

The big story of the day was Kassia and her new haircut. I left Kassia and Koby with a friend while I accompanied Aleks for his first two hours of the day. While she was at their house, Kassia and her friend Hannah decided to give each other haircuts. It was pretty minor compared to what I have seen other kids do. She and Hannah will be sporting the most interesting haircuts when preschool starts in two weeks!

Stacey

Sent: Wednesday, October 12, 2005
Subject: dream

Hi, Mom,

I was thinking about your dream about Grandma Hoffman on the way home. I thought it was interesting.

I remember a dream I had about two weeks before she passed. She was out on a boat ramp by the water wearing a dress. (The dress was out of place for the setting.) In the dream, she gave me a big hug and said, "Goodbye." It was a very intense dream—probably the most convincing evidence I have had of a supernatural being or connectedness. Don't ask me the color of the dress, I don't know if I dream in color.... do you?

Stacey

Sent: Friday, November 11, 2005
Subject: hi

Hi, Mom and Gary,

Thank you for sending me one of the invites to your opening. It is sooo cute. I visited Lesley yesterday, and everyone at the pharmacy was looking at the kids because they recognized the picture from your postcard. Lesley must have it up at work.

Aleks and I test for our next belts in Kyuki-do on Wednesday night. I am proud of Aleks. He has finally memorized his form and can do it with confidence.

Kassia drew us the story of *The Wizard of Oz* in her notebook this morning. It is really cool.

Koby has had some successes with his potty training over the last couple of days. He has been quite a character lately. He likes to be Aladar, who is a dinosaur in the dinosaur movie. When he is doing one of his characters, he calls me "Stacey." I guess he is not my little boy when he is Aladar.

Stacey

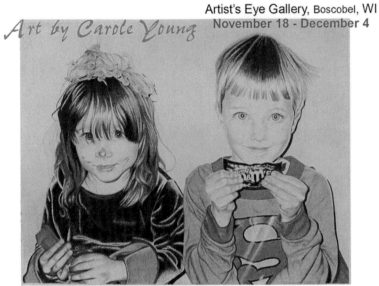

Art by Carole Young

Trick or Treat Inventory, 2005, colored pencil, 16" x 20"

In November 2005, Stacey and Tommy vacationed in Costa Rica. Grandma Carole and Grandpa Gary came from Boscobel to babysit and spend Thanksgiving with Aleks, Kassia and Jakoby. Following are excerpts from her memories of that trip.

Costa Rica, 2005, Nov. 21

Our flight to San Jose was flawless. We arrived in San Jose Costa Rica at 6:35—on schedule. From the plane, we entered a modern airport with familiar restaurants like Burger King and Schlotzsky's Deli (chuckle). We proceeded to the baggage claim as we waited patiently with other passengers for our luggage. The sound of dogs barking loudly on the premises was a little unsettling.

• • •

Once we were out of Sarchi, we climbed in elevation and entered rural Costa Rica. It was cloudy, foggy and beginning to rain. We could not appreciate the expanse of the landscape, but occasionally the fog would lift, and a mountain would appear beside us. It was clear enough to enjoy the views alongside the road. A wide variety of trees—palm, eucalyptus, etc. and plants. Everything was so green. The roadsides were lined with flowers of many types. The most common flower was impatiens. For miles, we saw these in all colors—red, purple, and pink.

• • •

Nov. 22

The night ahead was one of very little sleep. Fortunately for us, the skies cleared, and we had a full view of the volcano. Occasionally I would force myself to roll over and go back to sleep only to dream of the volcano erupting again and having to take a look. Tommy also had weird dreams about the volcano all night. Maybe it is impossible to sleep under such a power of nature. The most amazing thing to me is that you could actually hear the large rocks and boulders bouncing down the sides.

• • •

Nov. 23

We signed up for the morning hike, which was also included with our room rate. About twenty of us set off with the guides on a three-hour hike to explore the rainforest and lava beds in this pristine national forest. At the beginning of the hike, we were given the choice to traverse a small river barefoot or to step across on the rocks. We chose the rocks along with the majority of the group.

We entered the forest. Our guide spoke pretty good English through a heavy accent. The first thing he pointed out to us was some busy little ants. This long trail of ants wound its way up a vine on the tree and then down through the forest. Each ant was carrying a piece of leaf that was about five times its body size. At first, I dismissed this as something that was not very amazing. I struggled to understand the guide's English as he told the story about how these ants live for only seven days. They carry the leaves to feed the fungus which feeds their babies and the queen ant. This is their sole purpose in life, and they do this 24-hours-a day for six days non-stop. On the seventh day, they die. Then it hit me. I felt I was looking at an example of this precious web of life.

These ant's sole purpose on this planet was so clearly defined. I stared at the ants and then noticed the backdrop of the volcano which had just let out another one of its hissing sounds. Though familiar, this hissing sound always stopped our guide in his tracks. The potential of this volcano is to wipe out all of existence in a five-mile radius. It seemed that all there was to know was right in front of me. A totally amazing image not photographed but branded in my mind forever.

· · ·

Nov. 28

It was a trip of contrasts—safe and calm vs. dangerous, forest and city. I believe I thought that visiting the rainforest would change my life dramatically. Looking back, I can't say it did. I have a great respect for what is there and would even say I would be cautious about going there again. The human impact in this delicate place was easy to see, and every visitor does make an impact no matter how careful they are. It is an absolutely beautiful place where one can't help but to slow down and look at the little things—a butterfly waking up, a small plant that curls upon touching it, a flower that is white one day and purple the next. If I can remember to appreciate these little things and to look for the same kind of beauty in my surroundings in suburban Chicago, I think I have learned everything I need to from the rainforest—and I will never forget those ants!

Sent: Monday, November 28, 2005
Subject: back home

Mom and Gary,

We got in about 7 tonight. It was a fine flight back. We had lots of bonding with the kids until 9. I haven't even opened my suitcase. Plenty of time for that tomorrow.

Thanks again for your help. We had such a great time, and the kids seem like they did too! Tired now.

Stacey

Sent: Wednesday, December 07, 2005
Subject: Christmas prep

Hi, Mom,

I was just thinking about baking Christmas cookies. I have fond memories of making cookies with you. I have always been a little envious of Laurie living close to you and being able to share that tradition with you even in recent years. It would be fun if we could get together and make cookies together again.

Other holiday news: Aleks more or less explained he doesn't believe in Santa. It was a complicated story. Some kids at school told him Santa died and now parents have replaced Santa. Aleks came up with his own theory that Santa went down a chimney and got burned. Boo hoo! Aleks also said he started thinking this after Christmas last year.

I suppose he doesn't believe in the tooth fairy either. He pointed out that the pink index paper I wrote the fairy note on was from our office upstairs. I dug deep to find some paper he would not recognize. He is just too smart.

Love Stacey

CHAPTER 14
Mantra: "We Love Elgin"

Sent: Sunday, January 29, 2006
Subject: birthday fun

Hi, Mom and Gary,

We had a great day at the aquarium. My favorite part was seeing a giant sea turtle swimming by us in a large tank. It stopped in front of Koby and gave him a little birthday kiss. Of course, I did not have the camera ready. We saw the dolphin show, too. That is always fun.

The aquarium is really a nice place to appreciate the diversity we have on this planet—what a learning experience for the kids. Thanks again—it is nice we can still enjoy a Christmas gift from last year.

Stacey

Sent: Friday, February 24, 2006
Subject: morning coffee

Hi,

I just had to share this with you. I was all curled up in front of my morning coffee this morning when Aleks commented, "You look just like Aunt Laurie, Aunt Lesley, and Grandma Carole when you wake up and do that." He went on to say it was the way I had my knees curled up and was looking down at my coffee and just waking up. I thought it was funny. I am now working on my second cup and am getting my morning rolling. I am in an upright position at least.

Love, Stacey

Sent: Sunday, March 19, 2006
Subject: pancakes

Hi,

I thought you would like this one. I was struggling to make pancakes this morning. They were burning, sticking to the pan, and I hadn't had my coffee. I prepared a stack of about 10 pancakes. They weren't the best-looking pancakes, and they were slowly getting cold as I called the kids to the table.

Once the kids were seated, I retreated to a chair with newspaper and coffee in hand. I had barely sat down when I heard at least three complaints about the pancakes (burned, cold, not enough syrup). I reacted by saying, "Oh, come on, I tried so hard to make those pancakes. I don't want to hear you complain about them."

Kassia said, "Oh, Mom they are really good." Aleks then piped up and said, "I am trying hard to eat them...."

Stacey

Sent: Saturday, May 06, 2006
Subject: parade

Well, I did it. I twirled nunchucks in the Cinco de Mayo parade here today. What fun.

Aleks and Kassia paraded in their uniforms, too, and performed a couple of small demonstrations.

Stacey

Sent: Monday, June 12, 2006
Subject: survivor

Hi, Everyone,

Well, I survived the ropes course that was put together through our martial arts school. It really did not involve too many ropes. The games we played were a little like *Survivor*. Example: getting everyone in our group over a 12-foot wall with no rope—just some strong backs and arms, some interesting balancing beam exercises, getting all 15 of us in a 30 by 60-inch box crawling in from the bottom and out the top while crammed like sardines. I did not think the physical part of it was as difficult as the mental part and balancing. Most of the people in our group were in pretty good shape because of the martial arts. At least half of us were over 40. It must have done a number on me because the kids were tossing blankets on me as I curled up asleep on the sofa at 8 p.m. last night, and it took three lattes for me to get going today.

Stacey

Sent: Wednesday, July 19, 2006
Subject: power

Hi, Mom and Gary,

I think our power was restored just after 2 p.m. today. We are supposed to have more thunderstorms this evening. I hope they aren't nearly as eventful.

It was a great opportunity to clean the refrigerator out!

Tommy and I have also talked about living "off the grid" someday. Hmmmmm. I think we will want to have plenty of solar panels to back up our geothermal system. Two days was a good enough experiment for now.

Actually, it was nice. Without my computer and the kids without the TV, there was more quality time. Last night we played catch outside until we could no longer see, and then we came in and had a candle night.

Stacey

Sent: Tuesday, August 01, 2006
Subject: Re: Birthday

Hi,

The kids are looking forward to their visit. I thought we were going to have a busy week around here, and instead they are bored out of their minds.

They have been doing great in their swimming lessons. I think all have made significant progress. Aleks is dunking under all the way and is starting to swim a little. Kassia jumped off the diving board yesterday. Koby converted into a shark and would not come out of the water for me. I stood there helplessly fully clothed while he convinced me he had gills and needed to stay in the water to live. I tried to tempt him by saying we would go home and take a bath. He explained that the tub is not big enough. He needed lots and lots of water for his swimming. See you soon.

Love, Stacey

Sent: Wednesday, August 23, 2006
Subject: first day

Hello Everyone,

We did it. We survived another first day of school. This year was especially memorable as we saw Kassia off to her first day of kindergarten.

Tom and I woke at 6:00 a.m. to a BEEP BEEP BEEP. "What is that?" Tom said. I soon recognized that it was Aleks' Batman alarm clock being broadcast over the baby monitor. I managed to pull myself out of bed by 6:40. I proceeded down the stairs to find Aleks fully dressed, hair combed, with backpack on and ready to go. My only thought besides how handsome and grownup he looked was, "Are you really that anxious for the summer to end?" Kassia wasn't far behind. She had a jumpstart on her dressing by wearing her clothes the night before. (I made her change her underwear.)

As the years go on, I am getting a little more organized. I planned for the fact I had two kids going to school with a pile of school supplies, lunch money, lunches, special medications (Kassia), and packed the night before. This way we were able to have a warm breakfast, and I would not have to play drill sergeant to get everyone dressed. Other than Kassia pushing Koby down in an argument, the morning went smoothly. We did not have any glue spilling in backpacks this year.

The first casualty on the way to school was Koby falling down and skinning both of his knees. Fortunately, one of the required supplies for Aleks was a box of Band-Aids so we were fully prepared. Of course, the scrapes rendered Koby unable to walk, so I ended up carrying him the remaining four blocks to the school. This was fine. I needed the workout. What I did not need were the pools of sweat on my shirt. It was already a hot and humid day.

We arrived at the school and saw Aleks off to his second-grade line. Kassia could not wait to go stand in the kindergarten line. She pulled my arm, and we headed off in that direction. She looked so grown up in line with her denim skirt and black Hello Kitty backpack. She had her nails painted in rainbow colors and her hair braided for an added touch. The kindergartners all looked brave but a little bewildered wondering what was ahead for them. Kassia is almost the tallest in her class of 13. I repeat 13! The afternoon class only has 11. That is fantastic in a school district where class sizes of 30–35 are not out of the norm.

I spent the first hour of the morning in the kindergarten class. I wasn't much help with Koby, but I was able to socialize with some of the other parents. It was fun to watch the teacher get acquainted with the children. One poor little boy was having a terrible time. I felt bad for him but would not doubt he is the class clown by the end of the year. I watched Kassia complete her first assignment, a self-portrait. She finished the crayon drawing and proudly printed her name across the bottom, not forgetting how to make her kindergarten A's.

Next, we proceeded to the second-grade classroom. A very complicated school supply inventory was in progress. I was careful to be very thorough with Aleks' supplies. I did pretty good. Out of 25 required supplies, we were short one highlighter. The high point of Aleks' day was that he is in the same class as his best friend, Nathan. They were allowed to sit next to each other today. I predict that seating arrangement will last one week. They were already making dinosaur hand signals to each other in the time of my short visit. Aleks also has a small class. I counted 19.

The school day ended with Aleks taking a tumble on the way home. He was running full speed and managed to scrape the top of his hand, his hip, and his knee in one fall. I guess he won the award for the most Band-Aids needed. We celebrated the first day with Scooby-Doo push pops. Yippee!

Stacey

Sent: Monday, October 09, 2006
Subject: Hi, Mom and Gary,

Today we did a little shopping. I went to the thrift store and bought four pairs of jeans for between .80 and $1.20 each. A couple of pairs were very nice Levi's. What a steal! We also worked on Halloween costumes. Aleks settled on being a paleontologist (whew!), and we found him a really cool khaki vest. We also got boots, a belt, and khaki pants (under $10 for all!). My only job will be to write #1 Paleontologist on the back, and Aleks and I will work together on drawing a Utahraptor claw with fabric paint. That is a little more up my alley. We will also have to find some tools. Kassia will be the dinosaur/dragon, and Koby wants to be a ghost. They are being so easy on me. It will be nice not to spend $60 on costumes.

I better go make dinner. I haven't told Tommy I have kickboxing tonight. I should probably have things settled so he can watch Monday Night Football with the kids. We will talk to you soon!

Stacey

Sent: Thursday, October 26, 2006
Subject: that's my girl

Today my braided hair Kassia came home and told me that Lucas does not like braids. I asked her, "Did he tell you that?"

She said, "No, Noa (girl) told me that." Could this be a sign of a little competition? This Lucas boy seems very popular with the girls.

The best part was when I asked Kassia, "Does this mean you won't wear braids anymore?" She said sometimes she will and sometimes she won't. I guess that Lucas' opinion does not mean that much to her. That's my girl....

Stacey

Sent: Wednesday, November 01, 2006
Subject: Halloween

Hi, everyone,

Hope you all had a spooky nice Halloween. We had a great time. The kids were out for almost two hours last night. Kassia said her legs were tired when she got home. I don't know if it was the miles they put on or the truckload of candy that was dragging behind her when she got home

Koby pooped out early. Once he had a couple dozen pieces of candy, he was content to go home in the warm house and eat and eat and eat. Smart.

People go all out for Halloween here. I heard reports of the kids having to reach in a steamy trunk to get their candy. Another house had a live snake in the candy!

This morning, I estimate we have about 500 pieces of candy dumped in our dining room. Aleks was organizing piles. The following were his pile categories: 1. chocolate/crunchy candy, 2. hard candy, 3. chewy candy, and 4. non-candy (other). Next came an hour of negotiating and trading. I was not surprised when the trading was done that Aleks' pile was three times larger than everyone else's. (Kassia and Aleks went to all the same houses and should have had the same amount). I did not make a big deal of it because I will give them one more day and then the candy will be mine! Should I call the dentist now?

Love, Stacey

Sent: Thursday, November 02, 2006
Subject: Koby's observation

Hello,

We have been enjoying many little observations from Koby lately as he tries to figure out the world around him. One day he asked me, "Are we on the world?"

Last night we were out, and he was afraid of the night sky because it was really dark and black, not dark blue. He said it looked like space and not sky.

Today I got a chuckle. We were in the car, and he said, "There sure are a lot of Spanish people in this world." From his point of reference, that was probably a pretty accurate observation.

Stacey

Sent: Saturday, December 02, 2006
Subject: mishap

I am so excited about my date and fancy party tonight, but guess what.... I whacked the bridge of my nose with my car door and split it open leaving me with a half-inch cut down my nose. I think it is closing and healing, so I will skip the doctor and may have to face the fact that I may have a little scar.

Fortunately for me, the party is with a bunch of martial artists and not Tom's company party. I will just look like one of the gang.

Stacey

Sent: Monday, December 04, 2006
Subject: hi

Hi, Mom,

It is so cold today. We had a rough time getting to school. It was a difficult walk for Koby, and many sidewalks were not shoveled, so the wagon wasn't an option. I will take a sled to pull Koby when we go back this afternoon. The sun is out, so maybe it won't seem as cold.

We had a nice weekend. It was good getting out on Friday, but I think next time we put out $70 for a date we will go to the city and whoop it up. It wasn't our kind of party, and the food was OK but not excellent. It was fun dressing up, and I was happy I did not have to wear a Band-Aid on my nose like I did earlier in the day.

On Sunday, the kids and Tommy went to get a tree in the morning. The tree they got is cute and small. They chopped it down, so it is also very fresh. We put both electric trains around the base of the tree. The kids are very excited about that. We played Christmas music last night. The house is so cozy when it is decorated.

Stacey

Sent: Sunday, December 17, 2006
Subject: Santa

Hi, Everyone,

It was a nice night at the zoo last night. The zoo lights were beautiful. I did not wear my walking shoes, but we made it around to several exhibits before my feet were blistery and Koby kept falling down. We covered a lot of ground. I was dressed for a party and not a zoo trip. I thought the party was fine, too. They really catered to the kids. Tom did not think it was much of a company party. I guess face painting and magicians were not up his alley.

At the party, the kids got to sit on Santa's lap and tell him their wishes. I heard the children in front of us ask for iPod's and Nintendo stuff. I think my kids really threw Santa for a loop. First there was Koby who asked for a ghost. Second was Kassia, whose only request was a tiger toy. Lastly, there was Aleks who confessed he could not think of anything he wanted. (What happened to that long list of Utahraptor stuff he wanted?)

A busy weekend... On Friday, we dined at the Rainforest Cafe. Kassia's birthday request is the only thing that could get me within a five-mile radius of Woodfield Mall at the height of the shopping season. We survived it. In fact, we had so much fun we decided to go over to Build a Bear and make a little friend for her—a little snow leopard. She named it "Jaguar" and dressed it in a sparkly pink skirt and hoodie. She is worth every one of those 30 minutes in line that it took to bring her to life!

Look forward to seeing all of you on Christmas.

Love, Stacey

(A continuing conversation between Carole, Stacey, and Stacey's brother, Garret about the air quality in Boscobel from a polluting factory.)

From: Carole Young
Subject: yah scary

I would be hesitant and probably too cowardly to start a major campaign in Boscobel. Too many people depend on it for their living, and I don't want to end up with rocks through my window or the victim of a questionable accident and the postmortem heroine of a new movie.

Although I don't think we will make that direction a destination for our walks, I don't really know the overall impact on the air quality of Boscobel as a whole. Maybe the prevailing winds blow most of it to the east of us. And also, is it any more dangerous than living in a big city with exhaust fumes spewing out poisons? It is a shame we are poisoning ourselves on this planet.

Mom

Sent: Friday, February 23, 2007
Subject: Re: yah scary

I think it is good to be aware of, and I think you are right—it is everywhere and is much worse in some areas. There is plenty of fresh air in and around Boscobel.

One thing we can do is watch what we put into our own homes. People may be getting higher exposures of these chemicals in their homes with carpets, new sofas, paints, and adhesives. Exposure to these are persistent and don't change with the prevailing winds.

Stacey

Sent: Sunday, March 4, 2007
Subject: Article on how to offset your "carbon footprint" by planting trees

Here is a link to a site with info on your "carbon footprint."

It is a way for those who are concerned about the effects their lifestyle is having on the planet to get absolution from their polluting sins. Kind of like a Catholic confessional, but instead of alms or Hail Mary's, you plant trees or donate to people who help the environment.

Garret

Sent: Sunday, March 04, 2007
Subject: Re: Article on how to offset your "carbon footprint" by planting trees

Good website. Thank you for forwarding it, Garret. It's not a confessional but a new way of life that we all need to think about. We changed out all of the lightbulbs that we could to CFL's and saved at least $10 a month on electricity. We have been looking for ways to further reduce and calculated that our 18-year-old refrigerator is costing us $25 a month to run. That baby is out of here.

Tom and I attended a solar workshop this weekend. We are in need of a new water heater and are considering solar. The upfront costs are high, but there is a return on your costs after a period.

I've also found ways to simplify my shopping to once a week or so. Not only is it decreasing the amount I drive, but it makes life so much easier than running to the store every day or two. More time to do the things I enjoy.... I try to coordinate trips so I make a few stops with each trip out and do it when I am not with the kids. There's a lot more that I (we all can do). Thanks again.

Stacey

Sent: Wednesday, May 16, 2007

Hi, Mom and Gary,

Koby has been a little bit of a challenge in preschool lately. He only has four more days—hopefully the summer will bring some changes. He is gaining in many skills both social and academic. He copies the alphabet from those cards we got in Boscobel and writes his name. He has the most amazing questions about things right now. We were waiting for Kassia to go into the school at Lowrie the other morning, and he asked, "Why do we have a light-skinned family?" He is still really fascinated with Egypt but does not like to admit it.

Love, Stacey

Sent: Monday, July 23, 2007

Hi, Mom,

We had a good weekend. Tom did lots of yard work on Saturday. I got my hair done and did Kyuki-do class with the kids. At night, we went to an outdoor movie down by the river in the new park. They showed a sing-along version of *The Wizard of Oz*. It was fun. We brought some popcorn and drinks and spread out a blanket. The weather and sunset were perfect for the event.

On Sunday I went out and put my time in at the labyrinth. I had not been out in a couple of weeks—whew, the weeds are winning! That happens this time of year. I had plenty of help, so some progress was made.

Aleks is busy planning our Seattle trip. I am getting him involved in it as a way to keep him involved in writing, math, and reading. It will be a good little project. He is digging it so far. Talk to you soon.

Love, Stacey

Sent: Wednesday, August 15, 2007
Subject: hi from Seattle

Hi, everyone,

Our trip has been good so far. Our flight was on time. The kids were a little bored at times but were totally amazed at the sight of the Cascade Range (Mt. St. Helens, Mt. Hood, Mt. Adams, Mt. Rainier) upon our descent into the Sound. The only catastrophe was a bottle of spilled milk all over the inside of Aleks' carry-on. The itinerary he so carefully put together in a binder was soaked with milk. He took it pretty well, and we were able to salvage it.

We have been VERY active. We went to the market and aquarium yesterday. Basically, the kids were up from 4:10 a.m. until after 10 p.m. central time. It was a very full day for them. Koby had slept about two hours on the flight, so that helped.

We had to settle for a room on a lower floor of the hotel so that we would have enough beds for all of us. Amazingly, what was considered lower level of this hotel is the 17th floor. We have a clear view of the Space Needle, monorail, a little water, and mountains. I am looking out at a nice night city view as I type.

I went jogging this morning for about 2 miles along the Sound and through our old stomping grounds in Belltown. I visited the P-Patch community garden. It was hard to tell where my old spot was, but I saw some very mature lavender (bushes not plants!) and would have liked to believe they were the ones I planted.

Today we spent a couple of hours exploring the little shops in the market. The kids were fascinated with all the different stores. Two of the stores were Egypt imports. Koby was in heaven. He is having a little trouble with "Seattle food," though.

In the afternoon, we took a bus to the zoo. We walked so much today.

The Belltown neighborhood has progressed in quite a nice way. I went out to get some breakfast items for the kids tonight, and people were out on the street everywhere. There are many new outdoor cafes. One of the shopkeepers recognized me and said, "You are Tom's wife, right?" I was amazed. She was the Korean woman who owned the little grocery store below the Concept One Apartments where we lived 12 years ago.

Seattle is certainly tempting us with good times and good weather. We are repeating the mantra "We love Elgin! We LOVE ELGIN!" just in case we get some crazy ideas.

Love you all, Stacey

Sent: Friday, August 17, 2007
Subject: trip continued

Hi,

Well, you knew it was coming. The big meltdown occurred on Wednesday afternoon at the Boeing Flight Museum just after boarding the Concorde and Air Force One. It wasn't a pretty picture, Tommy shouting at the kids, me rolling my eyes, and the kids whirling around happily and then fighting the next moment.

Fortunately, we are able to regroup, and things have been uphill ever since.

On Wednesday we went to the Environmental Home Center. The CEO gave me a big tour of their new and expanding location. He tempted me by telling me I had a job if I want to move back. Unfortunately, their expansion plans don't include suburban Chicago right now.

Hope all is well there. We are still having fun.

Love, Stacey

Sent: Sunday, August 19, 2007
Subject: trip

Hi, everyone,

Everything is still going great. We got all our scheduled Seattle stops in. We took a long trip to Mt. Rainier today. It was a little cloudy up there, but I think the kids enjoyed it. We ran into rain and heavy traffic coming back into Seattle—imagine that.

We spent the evening in our old neighborhood. There has been a great deal of change. The kids remembered the children's hair salon in the Wallingford Center, but the toy store, burrito store, and children's clothing store were all gone. There was still a little train table in the hallway. It seemed very lonesome in there. The ice cream store down the street was also gone. It was replaced by a store that sells political buttons and banners. I wanted to tell Lesley there is a natural pharmacy in the Wallingford Center now. It looks like a nice store. I can't wait to tell her of some of the other changes. She knows that area well.

The block in front of our old house not only has a nice beer and wine store, they have added a vegetarian Thai restaurant and a chocolate store. I would be in real trouble if I still lived there.

We are off on a morning ferry. I will update if we can hook up, but we will be out in the rainy, rainy rainforest, so who knows what the internet service will be like. Hope all is well there. Good to hear from some of you, too!

Love, Stacey

Sent: Wednesday, October 03, 2007

Yes, Aleks does like math. While he was working on some problems from a workbook the other day, a bunch of kids came to the door, and he wanted to finish the math before going outside.

I was relieved today to have two little neighborhood skateboard punks come to the door and ask if Aleks wanted to play. He ran out the door and was tossing around a football with them in no time. We won't turn him into a total nerd.

Kassia has bells practice tonight, so we will go out to church. She had her first performance on Sunday and did just great after only three practices. She plays the F and E bells. I think she likes it a lot. They will perform "Aura Lee" on Music Sunday, November 11. I just realized they ring for the Christmas Eve service. We will have to stick to our usual plan for the holidays and come on Christmas Day.

I have to go. Koby wants me to find a hat for him so he can dress up like Elwood and sing "Sweet Home Chicago." Never a dull moment....

Stacey

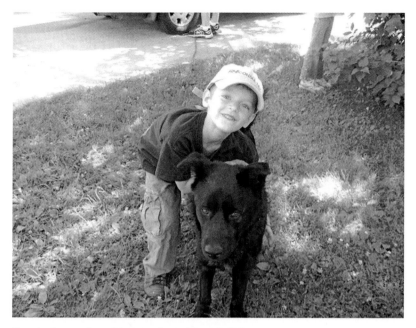

Sent: Saturday, November 10, 2007
Attach: IMG_2167.JPG; IMG_21 70.JPG
Subject: new family member

Meet Midnight, the newest member of the Reynolds/Lesiewicz family. He is 8 weeks old.

It was kind of a spontaneous move for us. The moment was right, and we had these adorable puppies placed in front of us. The kids are thrilled, and the dog has bonded beautifully.

He is a mixed breed, but from what we know, he is mostly a Keeshond. Look at these pictures. You can see why there was no resisting him!

Stacey

Sent: Thursday, December 20, 2007
Subject: trip

Hi, Mom and Gary,

We will plan on leaving before 10 a.m. on Christmas Day. We would like to stay two nights, leaving sometime on the 27th.

Tommy is mortified about bringing the dog to someone else's house He said, "We just don't do that." I convinced him that we will look into other options on the next trip.

On the way back from bells practice last night, Kassia posed some questions from the backseat. "So, is Santa real or is it someone else or is it you?"

I said, "Kassia! Don't you believe in Santa anymore?"

"Yeees (giggle, giggle)," was Kassia's response.

I said, "Do you think Mommy really has the time and money to get all those presents?" She seemed to think so. It should be a fun year.

Stacey

Sent: Wednesday, January 16, 2008
Subject: hi

Hi, Mom and Gary,

I have been taking the kids to Kyuki-do twice a week, and I have been going to around four classes a week. I got the paperwork this week to test for my brown belt—so watch out! I need to decide if I will test this month or wait. They expect a lot at this point. I have a vocabulary of about 150 Korean words, something I would not have expected to learn at this point in my life! I will have to break the board with a spinning hook kick or something crazy like that. Still one to two years to my black belt, so I have plenty more to learn.

I worked at the preschool today and am really proud of how Koby has settled down. It seems that he has taken a growth spurt physically and in maturity. Several people have commented on the change. I have noticed improvement at home, too. We are planning an Egypt birthday for him. I have two weeks to figure out how I am going to pull it off.

Kassia purchased a pink guitar with her Christmas money. I am hoping that she can take lessons someday. She's a cool little girl. Instead of running around worshipping Hannah Montana, she wants to get her own guitar.

I have to come up with something special for Tommy's b-day. I have Bunco that night, and he insists I go.

Stacey

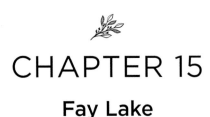

CHAPTER 15
Fay Lake

In July 2008, extended family members gathered "up north" in Crandon, Wisconsin, to attend the 50th wedding anniversary of Russell and Arlet Steel, Stacey's aunt and uncle. As she booked her own family's stay at Fay Lake Resort near there, she reminisced about the resort and past experiences there as a youngster.

August 1982—A family gathering convenes at Fay Lake on this mid-August weekend. Some have traveled far to get here. An extended family of grandparents, uncles, aunts, cousins, and siblings will spend the weekend fishing, swimming, and boating. It is the perfect setting for such a gathering. The trees are showing just a hint of the autumn colors that will come, a bit of yellow and orange among the deep greens. The sun shines, but the air has a hint of the fall crispness that will be descending on this place within a few weeks. This day on the lake will be marked by a special announcement. It is both a surprise and a blessing. Soon there will be a new member to our family. A baby is on the way. One of the cousins is expecting a child. She is very young, but the news is received with joy and acceptance by all. A close-knit celebrative feeling marks the news this weekend.

That was the second year my family visited Fay Lake. I was a teenager. There were moments when I did not appreciate this vacation with my family. I remember staring at the walls of my private bedroom in that little cabin. Even back then, the walls were a little crooked and cracked, the curtains faded. I remember thinking to myself, "What kind of place is this?" I felt imprisoned. I felt separated from my boyfriend. Back then, we did not have the internet or personal communication devices. A phone call to my boyfriend was dependent on the availability of a large number of quarters for the pay phone. It seemed to be a very large obstacle at that time. Finally, a postcard was delivered to me. My boyfriend had sent it! This positive affirmation was all I needed to enjoy the rest of my vacation, which at that time involved getting as much sun as possible and digging into the latest Danielle Steele novel. We did not worry about the sun in those days. We just slathered on the SPF 4 with a little baby oil and browned ourselves up. Looking back at my life back then, I was a little silly. Little did I know that I would look a little further and find the love of my life. How could I have been so blind as not to see the beauty or character or just enjoy the funkiness of this place? When did I learn to stand on my own? Soon I would be heading off to college, and eventually I would find my way. Although, it would be many years before I found out who I really am.

I've been thinking about that summer on the lake with the extended family. The women and the kids spent the day by the pool or running around the farmyard. The men took the boats out and fished. When the boats came in, they cleaned up the catch that would be part of the dinner. When the sun was out, we played outside. When it rained, I remember enjoying those board games, the laughter, the trickery, the fun.

We were all young and healthy. There was no illness or death lurking in the future of this bright shiny family. It seemed as if it would be this way forever, and these relaxing sun-filled days would never end. The night would wind down, and there would be a big dinner of fresh fish or grilled burgers. When it was time to clean up, we sang. We sang as we washed dishes just as we did at home. There was drinking. By the end of the night, at least one of the men had drank too much. It always ended happy, though, at least for now.

July 2008—Another family gathering was happening in the Northwoods, my aunt and uncle's 50th anniversary, and it has been decided we will make the trip. Tom has been in a phase of steady employment and has built up some vacation time. We decide to make the most of the trip and vacation in the Northwoods. I guess it is the happy family memories I was clinging to when I searched the internet and found the Fay Lake website.

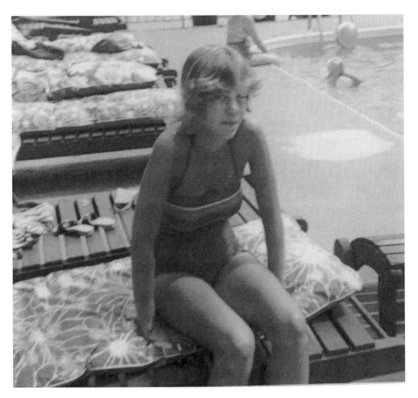

CHAPTER 16

Going Overboard on a Summer Schedule

Sent: Monday, April 28, 2008

I worked on a summer schedule, and I am really going overboard. They have all these creative camps around here for kids that I can't afford (robot building camp, art/nature camps, cooking camps, etc.). I decided our whole summer will be a camp, and we will have a theme each week with learning activities. I set it up around museum free days, our trips to Wisconsin, the kids' interests, and everything. It is really cool. Maybe I should have it published when it is all detailed.

I need to go down and give Tommy some attention. He is suffering from yet another migraine. Talk to you soon.

Stacey

Sent: Monday, May 05, 2008
Subject: hi again

Just to update, I took Koby in, and the doctor thought it was a pretty deep puncture wound. We need to swab it every night with peroxide (Daddy's job). It is gross because we actually need to stick the Q-tip into the boo-boo. He said it probably deserved a stitch or two last night, but then again it is a good thing it didn't get sewed up because sealing it tends to breed infection. He did not seem too overly worried about it. It should heal in 7–10 days. I called the amusement company but haven't gotten a call back. I am not going to get bent out of shape over a $73 doctor bill, but it is good to report in case something did happen, and it got worse and we had more expenses.

Midnight is having his little surgery. They will call when he is ready to be picked up. It is nice to get a little yardwork done without him barking, wondering what I am up to.

Stacey

Sent: Tuesday, May 06, 2008
Subject: Re: hi again

Koby's leg still looks good. Tommy is taking care of cleaning it at night and putting a "mummy wrap" on it. I am in charge of salving Midnight's surgical site. For some reason that creeps Tommy out, so I guess we have a fair trade.

Stacey

Sent: Saturday, June 14, 2008
Subject: Re: hi

I forgot to tell you about a couple of projects I am working on. Do you remember the dilapidated house at the end of our block? I am trying to get a movement started so that the city will buy it and develop it into a community house/community garden for our neighborhood. Maybe a private vendor could run a little coffee shop and gallery out of there. (Perhaps I could if they give me free rent for a million years.) I did a little rendition of the site and have been asked to present it at our meeting on Monday.

Our neighborhood also got a big grant to have houses researched for their historic value and plaqued. The city plaques houses of historic significance. Because of the above project, I am part of the Preservation Committee for our group and would be involved in this little project.

Stacey

Sent: Wednesday, August 13, 2008
Subject: Re: Lyme's Disease

Yikes, I hope you are feeling OK. I am glad you caught it early. We checked for ticks and rashes after our trip to Fay Lake. Everyone is looking good so far—even Midnight. I am amazed we found nothing after those days in the woods. It is getting more difficult to check the kids. They are starting to get so private.

Love, Stacey

CHAPTER 17
We Might Become Famous!

Sent: Thursday, August 28, 2008
Subject: Tom's surgery

I think they will be postponing Tom's knee surgery. The gastro doctor today said that he has a heart murmur. He has to see a cardiologist instead.

It's good they are finding this out—possible cause for his headaches (?) Mitral valve problem.

Stacey

Sent: Friday, August 29, 2008
Subject: heart

Hi, Mom and Gary,

Tom saw the cardiologist. He has a loud murmur in the left side between ventricles. The doctor said he may have had it for a long time—probably not a ticking time bomb—last weekend he was towing Koby up and down hills on the bicycle.

He will have an ECG and stress test next week. His blood pressure is fine. He is taking the doctor's advice of no strenuous exercise until they do the tests.

Stacey

Sent: Tuesday, September 02, 2008

Hi, Mom,

It's been a little crazy here. Day four of kindergarten... I had to pick Koby up off the sidewalk and carry him a block because he did not want to go to school. The teacher reports that Koby crumpled or rolled up any papers she tried to give him. He refused to participate. The rest of the week is Koby boot camp. We are taking away toys, no TV or computer, and he will go to Kyuki-do 2–3 times a week instead of once.

Tommy is anxiously waiting his appointment on Friday to get to the bottom of his health issues. He has been feeling chest discomfort— probably acid reflux like in the past, but now he is worried about chest pains. He wanted to go in today and have the tests done, but the doctor said he must wait. Apparently, the doctor is not worried at all. I don't like to see Tommy being a worrier. That is my job! He is the one always telling me I am being an obsessive freak.

We are watching Bush speak now. Tommy is getting more stressed out listening to all of these Republicans. How about that VP pick?

Stacey

Sent: Thursday, September 04, 2008

Tom has his doctor's appointment at 11 tomorrow. I think it will be fine. It will be good to know. The waiting has been intense.

Koby seemed to be happier today after kindergarten. He met a girl named Kelly. He asked me if I saw her come out today. "She was the one with the ponytail," he said. He wants to invite her over for a play date and wishes to dress up for the occasion. He asked if he could wear a black top hat. His friends are now Kayden, Jamarian, and Kelly. He wants to meet two more girls so there is an even split. So much for learning the numbers and alphabet—he wants to meet some girls!

Listening to McCain now. He's a little boring compared to Palin.

Love, Stacey

Sent: Sunday, September 07, 2008

Today we had a little party for Grandma Rose who turned 96 this week. After our little party, Grandma Robin watched the kids, and Tommy and I went for a bike ride. You don't have to worry about that guy.... I had a hard time keeping up with him towards the end, especially on the hill coming up from the river. We went 6 miles to West Dundee, had a beer at the brew pub, and then came back for a total of 12 miles. What a beautiful day. It brought back memories of our rides in Seattle. That trail is such a nice amenity.

Stacey

Sent: Thursday, October 09, 2008
Subject: Tommy's surgery

Hi,

Tommy's surgery went fine today. It was an ACL rebuild and a repair to one of the tendons. We were able to leave the hospital at 1:30 today—less than four hours after his surgery started. Amazing huh? The other amazing thing is he was able to walk to the bathroom without crutches before leaving the hospital.

He has been taking it easy at home. He has an ice compression machine that we run every hour, and he is enjoying the benefit of his medications and is sleeping right now.

Stacey

Sent: Sunday, November 02, 2008
Subject: famous grandchildren

Hello,

Well you might have some famous grandchildren after tomorrow. A former neighbor of ours is a marketing person and just pulled together a big ad campaign for CVS/Caremart. They are doing a photo shoot, and her proposal suggested they use people from the community instead of professional models to highlight diversity and save costs. She asked if we would be interested, and I went along with it after she assured me it was a safe and secure thing to do. I wanted to help her out, too, because she has had a difficult couple of months and has a lot on her plate. They selected us after a shoot we did on Thursday. Tomorrow we have to go for a two-hour photo shoot. I get to do it, too. She said I might be pouring orange juice in one and may have a teenager in addition to my kids. Eeeeh gads!

I got the kids all cleaned up tonight and will pack up some outfits tomorrow. We will go after school. They will look cute no matter what. I am a little less sure about myself. It has been a stressful couple of weeks, and I am already three weeks overdue for my haircut and color. Maybe I will get to pose in the healthcare ad as the woman with influenza or an allergy attack or something. We will get $400, so maybe I can go get a fresh lipstick for the occasion. Time to watch *Desperate Housewives*.

Love, Stacey

Sent: Monday, November 03, 2008
Subject: Re: famous grandchildren

Just got done with the shoot. I was a little more of a participant than I thought I would be. It was a very interesting process—a makeup artist, the whole bit. Aleks and Kassia want to make a career of it. They thought it was a much easier way of earning $100 than raking leaves.

I think it is very likely we will be featured in the next CVS pharmacy brochure.

I saw one shot of Aleks posing with a soccer ball with some other boys. It looked very good, like it belonged in a catalog. Tommy is grumpy because he did not get to do it. He could not get in for the preliminary shots we took last week. I had to have a substitute husband in the family shot. He wasn't nearly as good-looking, though.

Glad you don't think I am a horrible mom for pimping out my kids for $400. I was thinking it would be Christmas money, but they want to put it in their savings accounts. I think that would be good. They earned it. Talk to you soon!

Stacey

Sent: Monday, December 08, 2008
Subject: hi

Hi Mom,

Tom just walked in the door. I haven't had a chance to talk to him, but it sounds like he had a good day in Chicago. He has three new leads—two of which he thought were good.

He has a modeling job tomorrow. He will model as a doctor for $100. That makes us all famous and will put a little extra money in our pockets.

We decided yesterday that the two of us will start a business. It all came together, and I think we have found a good combination of our talent, networks, and passions. We want to start some kind of energy audit business, maybe a "not-for-profit" along with a "for-profit" consulting business. It is something that we can chew away at over the next year. He can still find a full-time job with insurance, and we can work on this in all of our spare time. I think it would be in line with what people need and where our country is headed and where future investment and grants might be. I know a priority of Obama is to make our schools, government offices, and businesses more energy-efficient.

We have a lot to learn and have found there are classes offered on the subject. We are lucky to have a good community college here in Elgin.

Stacey

Sent: Monday, December 15, 2008
Subject: Aleks' story

Aleks and I were doing his last-minute backpack check this morning, and he mentioned he had a note from the library indicating he had to pay a fine for a damaged book.

I pulled it out thinking maybe it would be $4 or $5 for a mark or loose binding. I was surprised to see a $20 fine and naturally was a little upset.

Of course, I went into a little bit of a rant and asked, "What could have possibly happened to that book to require a $20 fine?" (The famous "I don't know" shrug followed.)

By then, Aleks was choking back tears as I went in the kitchen to show it to Tommy. As I entered the kitchen, I heard a mumble from behind saying, "Maybe it was the banana."

Mystery solved. The moral of the story is never use a banana as a bookmark.

The joke at our house now is if there is somewhere we need to spread the blame—maybe it was the banana.

Stacey

Stacey and Tommy were married December 31, 1992, on the beach at Ocho Rios, Jamaica. Her mother, Carole; stepfather, Gary; and sisters, Laurie and Lesley, flew to Jamaica to attend the wedding.

From: Gary Young
Sent: Wednesday, December 31, 2008
Subject: Happy Anniversary!

Wishing you two the best on your special day. I remember most of that day, but the groom got his best man pretty foggy on rum. So, my memories are a wonderfully mellow picture of paradise in the tropics.

Love, Gary

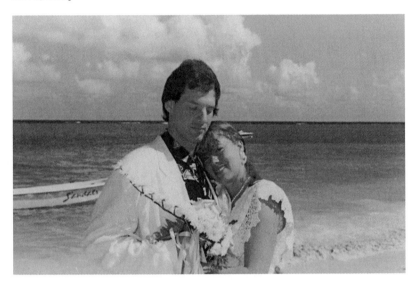

Sent: Wednesday, December 31, 2008
Subject: Re: Happy Anniversary!

Thanks!

We watched the videotape of the ceremony for the first time in many years. It was the first time the kids had seen it. Kassia seemed to enjoy it. Aleks was bored and only commented that he noticed the tape lasted exactly 30 minutes. Koby had some things to say. I could tell he was being very careful when he said, "I sort of recognize the eyes on it." (Meaning the bodies and hair have changed a bit.) And, "Mom, was it in the olden days? Cause it kind of looks like the olden days."

Well, 16 years have passed, but we all still have that sparkle, right?

Stacey

Sent: Tuesday, February 10, 2009
Subject: Re: Hi

Hi,

Thanks for the e-mail. It sounds like you had a busy day/week so far.

For the Facebook thing, I don't know if it is the greatest way for family members to communicate. Some people make multiple entries during the day, and you can pretty much follow everything they do. You can also find out what their favorite books are, what groups they are a fan of, etc. I am conflicted about being that public about things, even though the only ones that view my profile are friends. I'm warming up to it, though. I do not make many entries, so I am a pretty boring Facebooker. I have a small photo album that my friends can view. It is nice to be able to share photos that way.

Love, Stacey

Twenty-five random things about me.
Facebook, February 14, 2009

1. In my 44 years, I have called 19 places "home." My second longest home is my present home of 5.5 years—after my childhood home of 7.5 years. I have a strong connection to that place in spite of this.

2. Tommy and I have been together 26 years, and he still surprises me sometimes.

3. My hometown is a very small town in southwest Wisconsin. The "Turkey Hunting Capital of Wisconsin" and the "Birthplace of the Gideon Bible."

4. Tommy and I were married on a beach in Jamaica. It started to rain as we began our vows. To this day, I think it was a good omen and not bad. We spent three weeks exploring the island.

5. I do not have the capacity to be bored. There is always something to do, to look at or think about, and sometimes "nothing" is nice.

6. I hate traffic, shopping, malls, and big box stores. They sap the life out of me, and I avoid them as much as possible.

7. I wake up crabby most mornings. Tommy has adapted and makes me lattes and mochas. This along with his usual morning cheeriness brings light to the start of my day.

8. Eleven years ago, on this day, Tommy and I were driving around the deserts of southern Morocco in a rental car. A beautiful place and beautiful people. Speaking to the checkpoint guards in my very limited French was intimidating.

9. I am a very private person, so these notes are a strange thing for me to do.

10. 1995 was a sad year for me. I lost my dad and grandma, and Jerry Garcia died. In fact, I was on my way to my grandma's wake when I found out Jerry died. A sad day indeed!

11. For the second time in my life, I am months away from getting my black belt. This time I am going all the way!

12. My primary vices are red wine and dark chocolate. Fortunately for me, both are heart healthy in moderation.

13. I completed the Seattle to Portland bike ride twice. That is 200 miles in two days.

14. I never let my guard down—never. OK, some of my Kyuki-do (martial arts) friends who have managed to "slip one in" will disagree.

15. I was once alone on an elevator with Alex Rodriguez. We said "hi" to each other. I was breathless.

16. I have been married to a guy with very long hair, a guy with blue hair, and a guy with no hair. Fortunately for me, they have all been the same man.

17. Natural childbirth (no drugs), all three! Oh, I did cave in after 21 hours of labor on the first one, but I think it counts, doesn't it?

18. I'm not being obnoxious when I think my kids are smart and perfect. I just love them!

19. Tommy and I watched the last sunset of the 20th century on a beach in Hawaii. We said goodbye to 1999 much later than most people on the planet.

20. My goal in life is to be part of the solution and not part of the problem.

21. I've been some form of vegetarian for 23 years but still sneak pepperoni from my kids' pizza occasionally.

22. I am a sod warrior. I hope to dig up most of the grass in my yard within the next five years. My veggie garden and native prairie garden keep getting bigger and bigger,

23. My activist spirit started back in '73 (third grade) when I wrote to President Nixon asking him to stop the war. He responded with a form letter and a beautiful black and white picture of the president and first lady.

24. In '86, I went from a job interview straight to a Dead show. It was such a liberating feeling taking off that seafoam green business suit and heels and putting on sandals and tie dye. I should have followed my heart back then... or maybe not.

25. I once did interior design work for the Hilton's. You would never know it by looking at my house.

Sent: Friday, February 20, 2009
Subject: party at the Reynolds/Lesiewicz house

Hi,

Tommy got the job! He will be receiving an offer letter on Monday.

He starts next week sometime... similar to his other job—a few steps closer to the train station—more commercial in focus, a little less public sector. We are happy, relieved, and ready to party in a snowstorm tonight!

Stacey

Sent: Monday, February 23, 2009
Subject: my boy

Hi, Grandma and Grandpa,

Koby has been doing great at school, and we were aiming for a "grand slam" today—all stars three days in a row.

We had a little talk last week about teasing little girls. Apparently, he and another were calling a little girl a "name." At the time of the talk, I suggested that instead he say "hi" to her and maybe even say something nice. My suggestion was to say that her hair looked nice or that he liked her sweater.

I think he took my advice but perhaps added a little exuberance. Today he got in trouble for calling some girls "hot." Do you think I set him up for trouble?

Stacey

Sent: Thursday, March 05, 2009
Subject: Re: Hi

Hi, Mom,

Nice to hear from you!

It was a great day to be out. I have some daffodil buds peeking out of the ground on the south side of the house. I was very excited to see that.

I had another one of my marathon days. I am in the middle of a new fundraiser kickoff. I assembled 450 brochure packets this week, baked cookies, pitched the fundraiser at tonight's PTA meeting, and tomorrow I will do the intro for the kickoff assembly and make sure all of the teachers get their packets. I figure I walked about two miles today (as I do most), taking the kids to school and a 30-minute dog walk. Between walks, I managed to squeeze in a pretty tough Kyuki-do workout. It's now 8:30, and I am feeling very, very tired!

Tommy will be late tonight. His company had their annual Bowling and Billiards gathering tonight. It sounds like a fun place to work! So far, I think he likes it, and he is very happy to be out of the house and into a routine again.

On Sunday, we are meeting with another couple in Chicago to discuss the possibility of Tommy and me working with them to sell solar water heating systems—probably to businesses. It could be an interesting venture.

Love, Stacey

Sent: Saturday, March 07, 2009
Subject: hi

Hi, Mom,

We had a pretty lazy day around here. I went to the engagement party solo. Tommy stayed home with the kids. It was a very nice party with terrific food, and it was my first female couple engagement party! I got home from the party and everyone was waiting for me to make dinner. I thought I had stayed long enough for them to figure out that one for themselves! Tommy quickly made a dinner of mashed potatoes, nachos, and popcorn.

I have a little cleaning to do tomorrow before church. I think both Robin and Rose will be here with the kids while we buzz into the city. I am excited about talking to these people about the solar business. It sounds like something we would both have our hearts into that I can work on from home, mostly.

Love, Stacey

From: Carole Young
Sent: Sunday, March 8, 2009
Subject: Re: hi

Mashed potatoes, nachos and popcorn???? Hhhmmmm.

Hope you have fun today!

Mom

Sent: Monday, March 09, 2009
Subject: Re: hi

Hi, Mom,

Our meeting yesterday was nice/fun. The traffic was bad getting into the city because of the rain. We saw a total of four accidents. We ate at a nice little Thai restaurant. It was good to be in the city again.

It sounds like we are "in" as far as working on building a business with this couple. Nothing to lose and plenty of possibility! We are meeting again in two weeks to discuss the next steps. In the meantime, I may be visiting a solar collector factory in Chicago with them. Already I am marking my calendar for some upcoming events. It looks like we will be heading up to the Stevens Point area on June 20th for the Midwest Renewable Energy Fair.

Other than that, we are looking into some online classes. Our community college now offers several online classes in green technology. They are quite expensive but get you prepared for certification exams. I would have to sign up this month for a series of classes that begin in April.

Our first project might be to figure out how to get one of these installed on our house. If we can figure out a way to get lending (ha ha), apply for the government incentives, and work our way through the process, we will be prepared to sell to others. How are you? How's the painting coming?

Stacey

Sent: Friday, March 20, 2009

Hi, Mom,

Today was the last day of school before spring break. It was a little strange. Tommy stayed home from work because he had chest pains. He actually went to the hospital where they monitored him for a bit. His blood pressure was high when he went in, and they gave him a one-time dose of medication for that. Everything else checked out fine. He is scheduled for another routine stress test in two weeks, so I guess he will be seeing his cardiologist anyway.

We are not going to sleep in boxes tomorrow night. Quite a number of people from our church and area churches will be. Koby and Kassia both have coughs, so I was thinking we would sleep inside. Then it seemed a little pointless since we haven't gathered any pledges, and I don't have money for a personal donation. Aleks seemed a little disappointed when I mentioned it tonight. I think he wanted to sleep in the car. We will go and help with the soup kitchen, and the kids will watch a movie and listen to a church member who has experienced homelessness. I think there will be a good lesson without the discomfort of sleeping in the cold.

Koby will be testing for his yellow belt tomorrow, too. I am proud of how far he has come. He is excited because he will break a board. I will try to get a decent picture.

Love, Stacey

Sent: Saturday, March 21, 2009

Guess we might be sleeping in boxes or the car after all. I won't take Koby—his cough is too bad. The other kids REALLY want to do it and are willing to scrape together some of their allowance money towards the cause. Aleks was almost in tears when I told him we weren't going to do it this morning. It will be one to add to the memory book....

Stacey

Sent: Sunday, March 22, 2009
Subject: a nice night in the car

Mom and Gary,

We survived our "night out." We had an adequate turn out. It was definitely a kid-driven event with most of the Cardboard City residents between 6 and 12 years old along with the weary parents they dragged along.

We slept in the back of the car. The kids said they were warm. I would not say I was warm, but I have been colder camping in the summer unprepared. My complaint was sleeping on a hard surface. I was constantly tossing and turning with sore hips. Every time I turned, I had to make sure the blankets came with me. Can't imagine what it would be to sleep like that every night, and we had it good... just steps from the bathroom and a not-so-warm building, breakfast in the morning, and a drive home for a latte and warm bath.

Love, Stacey

Sent: Tuesday, April 28, 2009
Subject: hi

Hi, Mom,

I tested for my black stripe. Boy, did I work hard for that! It was quite a workout. I had to perform 11 forms (average 33 movements each). The finale for the night was a "speed break." I had to hold the board with one hand and break it with the other. I broke it on the second try. My hand is a little black and blue. Now I will work this summer to train for my black belt. The test is Nov. 5th.

I was very tired and sore today from the test (it was a 1.5-hour workout), but I still got some walking in—down to the school four times today plus a dog walk.

Love, Stacey

Sent: Thursday, April 30, 2009
Subject: hi

Hi, Mom,

Spent the morning shopping for groceries in the pouring rain.

I haven't been feeling great this week. I never totally recuperated from my workout on Monday. I think I have swine flu minus the sore throat and coughing. I did not feel like eating dinner last night and was happy with two pieces of watermelon. I was not hungry for breakfast this morning. My energy is up a little this afternoon, and I got the groceries put away and the house picked up.

The flu is getting closer to home as I look at news reports and talk to people. Cases are beginning to dot our county. Kassia's teacher was severely ill this week and was hospitalized in Chicago for the flu. Don't know if she was tested for swine flu, but I guess she was very dehydrated, which is serious with her transplant issues. She is home now, which is very good. Aleks said the father of one of his classmates is being tested for swine flu (maybe a story, maybe true).

I got grossed out at Kyuki-do last night because a kid was hacking away and did not look very energetic. When my kids came off the mat, I pointed to the hand sanitizer, which they always have available, and had them put it on right away. It doesn't help if there was coughing in the air, though. I think we will go "light" on classes until we know how widespread the flu is.

I made sure we had a stock of easy dinners, fever medicines, Kleenex, soap, and toilet paper. That is about all we can do at this point. The kids got that bad flu in January 2004. I remember what that was like—scary—but there was an end to it after a week of constant Ibuprofen doses, cool baths, popsicles, and lots of TV and sofa time.

Love, Stacey

Sent: Saturday, May 02, 2009
Subject: oink

Just when I thought this whole swine flu thing was going to go away, they closed our high school until next Friday because of a probable case. Larkin High is where we went for Kassia's concert on Thursday night. Oh, my!!! We are now exposed....

I believe I just saw my first masked person in Elgin. I heard some retail clerks in the area were wearing them. This was a high school-aged girl standing out on Moseley Street talking to someone with a bandana around her mouth and nose. Maybe she was just going for a gangster look.

Stacey

Sent: Saturday, May 09, 2009

Hi, Mom,

We had our long-anticipated garage sale today. I would say it was very busy. It helped that it was a street wide event—a real traffic stopper.

The results... $180, lots of happy faces, one mean racist customer spewing bad things about illegal aliens (around at least three Hispanic families), some big plastic toys that did not end up in the landfill, a clean garage, a slightly sunburned face, and a trip to Goodwill. The biggest surprise was the bicycle with no pedals sold.

In other news this week, Tommy had his six-month heart checkup, and everything looked good after a comprehensive three-hour exam. His blood pressure was high when he arrived, but they did not have much to say about that. He is waiting for a call to make sure he can go on his 100-mile bike trip and start martial arts. I think they will say "go for it."

Love, Stacey

Sent: Wednesday, August 12, 2009
Subject: job

I have a job! It is just a little job, but in this day and age to go from a whim and inquiry one day to the next day being hired, that's pretty good.

It isn't real exciting and is something I would not have expected doing.

I will be a lunch/playground supervisor at Lowrie two hours per day. I think it is $12 an hour. I will be equipped with whistle, nametag, and a deck of beaver tails.

My day will be split in half, and I will have 1 1/2 hours on each side to work on energy audit and Natural Dynamics stuff. Looks like I will be walking back and forth between home and school as much as last year.

A little extra money would not be a bad thing right now. Hopefully the kids won't eat me alive.

Stacey

Sent: Thursday, October 08, 2009
Subject: adventures of a lunch mom

Hi, Mom,

Just when I thought I had a handle on those third-graders, all hell breaks loose! That may be an exaggeration, but it has been a fun couple of days. Yesterday was going smoothly. It was a beautiful day, and the gym teacher had put out soccer equipment, so the kids were allowed to play. They had a great game and enjoyed themselves. After 20 minutes, we lined up and the kids were soon in the lunchroom preparing to eat their delicious chicken patties with ketchup and salad. The kids were about halfway into their lunch and were being reasonably quiet. Suddenly I felt a splat on the back of my head and turned around. The table in front of me had about five kids splattered in ketchup. Fingers pointed, and the accused was a beautiful little girl at the end of the table. Another girl showed me how the girl had made the ketchup splat with her hand, obviously smacking it with a great deal of force. I walked over to the girl and pointed out that her actions were wrong and had made quite a mess. She smiled, not completely realizing the consequence of her actions. One little boy was crying. He had ketchup in his eye. Naturally there was a stir among the tables as I gathered some napkins for the victims.

Today was a rainy day. We had indoor recess in the classrooms. My first group was a dream, and I rewarded them with a class beaver tail. For the second half of my shift, I walked up the stairs to the 3rd-grade room with some trepidation. I could already hear noise and running around before I got to the door, so I noted they are probably quite a handful for their teacher, too. He quickly left. About half the class was busy with quiet activities—nice! However, there was a large group of boys who seemed to have nothing to do. They wandered around chasing each other, basically obeying me if I asked them not to push, run, or to go sit at their desk.

Tom has a Citizen Action Committee for the school district tonight. It was announced this week that the district will be $54 million in debt by June, and that they need to make some cuts, layoffs, probably teachers and aides this time—possibly before year end.

Stacey

Sent: Sunday, November 08, 2009
Subject: Re: Home?

Got home at about 6:30 this evening. Weekend was great. Quote from Tommy a couple of minutes ago, "I think that was the funnest weekend our family has had in a long time."

Survived the black belt test... pictures to follow. Fortunately, some friends with much better cameras have promised some pictures.

Love Stacey the black belt—Hi-yah!

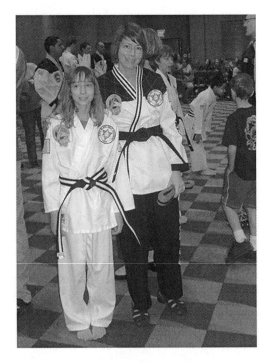

Sent: Wednesday, December 16, 2009
Subject: hello

Hi, Mom and Gary,

I wanted to let you know that Kassia got her present and is very happy. We will plan a shopping trip in the very near future.

We had a little family party last night. She opened her presents. We then went to the Colonial Cafe. When we got home, we watched her new Hannah Montana movie. After the movie, we tried to choke down the cherry cake that I made with pink frosting. I don't know if it was the flavor or the full bellies, but it was not very popular. While we were out, Midnight ate the beautiful plate of Christmas cookies on the table (my gift from the staff at the school). He hid behind the chair when we got home, overcome with guilt. Naughty dog!

I started the excavation of Kassia's room today in preparation for the sleepover. That girl sure does like to create! She loves to take boxes and create wonderful things. Unfortunately, her room cannot hold these creations forever. Wow, have I got my work cut out over the next three days....

Tommy is working today. He's got a company laptop, and we were all invited to Friday's Christmas party. Hopefully that full-time job offer will be coming soon!

He has an appointment on January 12 with the surgeon at Northwestern Hospital. We will know more about his surgery then. I will talk to you soon.

Love Stacey

Sent: Sunday, December 20, 2009
Subject: Re: Christmas

Hi,

Thanks for the update. I am in the middle of serving six little girls breakfast! Lights were out about midnight. They were up at 6 a.m.

We will have to keep our eye on the weather for Christmas. Looks like another big one is headed this way.

Stacey

CHAPTER 18
No Matter What, Mom, I'm Happy

Carole

"No matter what, Mom, I'm happy." These were Stacey's words as she called to break the news to me in January 2010. She had been diagnosed with stage 4 colon cancer.

Two months earlier, in November, she had earned her Black Belt in Kyuki-do and, also that month, gotten a clean bill of health from her general practitioner at her yearly physical. Continuing symptoms, which the doctor had dismissed early as caused by a non-threatening and common affliction, finally prompted the doctor to order a colonoscopy. Fifty is the routine age they are recommended. She was 45. They found, she said, what the surgeon described as an "angry mass." It was cancer, and a follow-up CAT scan revealed it had spread to her liver and lungs.

Husband Tommy was, at the same time, looking for permanent employment in the IT industry and prepping for open heart surgery.

There is no family history of colon cancer.

Stacey had been a vegetarian for years and bought organic whenever possible. She was a non-smoker, enjoyed an occasional beer or glass of wine, and was very physically active. Her years in Seattle were spent working in a "green industry," and she prided herself on a "chemical-free" home.

Sent: Monday, January 11, 2010
Subject: update

We are on a waiting list for appointments at University of Chicago for Tuesday and Thursday this week. I have an appointment scheduled for sure next Tuesday.

I still have an appointment with the surgeon here in Elgin tomorrow, although most are saying that chemo should come before surgery.

We told the kids, and they seem to be doing OK. They are such strong, loving children!

Still don't know what would be the best time if you wanted to come help. I am hoping we have some activity late next week—never thought I'd be anxious about a hospital visit. I am ready to get started in this fight.

Love Stacey

Sent: Tuesday, January 12, 2010
Subject: she's pierced!

Hi, Mom,

We got Kassia's ears pierced today. She looks pretty cool in her earrings and her new Justice for Girls outfit (we spent the gift card on Sunday).

Tom's appointment went well today. They do not have a surgery date. They are fairly flexible depending on our needs. We will find a time that works well with my treatments. More will be known next week. I think he is leaning towards having the surgery soon. They are giving him good odds of a quicker than normal recovery because of his physical condition. If I was to predict when he might be having It,

I would say in two or three weeks. It seems like that would be a good time for you to come depending on your schedule.

They are 98% sure they will not have to do a valve replacement—only a repair.

He is expected to be in the hospital (Northwestern Memorial) one week.

Full recovery in six weeks. After the recovery, he can return to light exercise and all normal activities. He cannot drive for three weeks after the surgery.

He can start working by computer once he is out of the ICU. They expect him to be there one day. The company he has been working for is very flexible and allows him to work from home.

Not much else new. I spent the day doing the usual stuff (walks to school, dog walks). I spent quite a bit of time on the phone and the computer doing research. Tom and I both crashed and took a nap when Janet took the kids to her house for dinner. That was very nice.

Love Stacey

Sent: Thursday, January 14, 2010
Subject: update

Hello, everyone,

I had a couple of doctor's appointments and feel like we fell into the hands of a couple of great doctors right here in Elgin—very warm and positive, and from what I hear, they come highly recommended.

We are still going to University of Chicago Hospital on Tuesday to see what they have to say.

On Monday, I will be having a minor surgical procedure at 1:30. They will put in a port so it can be used as an IV tube and can be used for blood draws, etc. Less needles—yeah! The procedure will only take an hour, and I can go home.

I did manage to squeeze a martial arts class in between doctor's appointments today. :) It was hard, especially after a large blood draw earlier, but I feel better afterwards. Tom joined me as he was approved to do light aerobic exercise.

It looks like I will be starting treatments middle of next week. If I do them in Elgin, I will be going in and out of their office for treatments and will also have a pump to administer the stuff while I am at home. Tom will probably have his surgery in two or three weeks.

Tomorrow is dentist day for me and the kids. Tom needs to go before they will do his surgery as well. Oh, these insurance companies are going to love us! I will keep you posted. Love to all, Stacey

Sent: Saturday, January 16, 2010
Subject: Re: Hi

Tommy had an interesting day. He went to talk to the company he has been working with to see when they could officially bring him on board. They continue to work on a plan to hire him and are very understanding and sympathetic of our current situation.

Lazy day today. I just have about two or three things on my to-do list.

Love Stacey

From: Thomas Lesiewicz
Sent: Monday, January 18, 2010
Subject: Stacey's surgery today

Hi,

Stacey is sleeping nicely. She had a long day. She had the Medi-port and a stent for her colon tumor. It started an hour and a half late, and her post-surgery recovery took a little longer, but the surgery went well.

Tomorrow we go to University of Chicago Hospital for our second opinion. Probably chemo on Wednesday. Wish her luck. Meditate. Pray. Light incense. Sacrifice a tofu chicken. The battle is starting this week.

If she's out of it from time to time, I'll try to keep you up to date. You can always call me anytime on my cell or email me if you ever want to reach me. I always have my Blackberry with me, and Stacey rarely has her cell phone with her. Thank you, tml

Sent: Monday, February 01, 2010
Subject: Re: Hi

Hi, Mom,

I enjoyed the visit, too, and yes, you were a very big help.

Janet came over and brought me some books and CD's. She was worried I would be bored during my treatment. I thought that was really nice, although I don't think boredom will be a problem. I think I said once that I do not have the capacity to be bored. I've got Tommy's iPod. I can bring the laptop. Plenty of books to read. Kassia and I started knitting again. Motivational tapes to listen to. Writing (?) Etc. Etc.

Stacey

Sent: Wednesday, February 03, 2010
Subject: hi

Hi, Mom,

Treatment went fine today. Tommy let me use his iPod. It is wonderful. I can download music, podcasts, motivational speakers, check e-mail, Facebook, browse internet. I enjoyed music today while reading.

My blood counts are low now (they checked them today before treatment). They were just at the threshold where he would postpone treatment. He recommended we do the treatment, and then they will give me a shot for a boost tomorrow. Now is when I will have to start watching GERMS. He chuckled when I said I had a sick coughing boy home for two days this week. Not a big worry. I am sure I will be going in for those 45-minute pin pricks often now.

Love Stacey

Sent: Wed, February 10, 2010
Subject: RE: hi

Did you feel the earthquake? Mom

Wednesday, February 10, 2010
Subject: Re: hi

Yes, we definitely did. Tommy and I both shot up out of bed and knew what it was. It was jolting and you could hear the rumble. Kassia woke up too.

I went downstairs and turned on the TV and no reports. Got my laptop out and people were already twittering about it.

They just changed the epicenter to Gilberts, Illinois. Very close to us. That is right around the Country Inn and Suites you stay at. Five or six miles from here?

The Geological Society says they do not know much about/haven't studied fault lines in our area. Great. I was leery about living on fault lines in Seattle. A little excitement to start the day.

Stacey

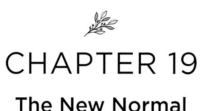

CHAPTER 19
The New Normal

Stacey received a Mayor's Award for researching the background of homes in her neighborhood that then became eligible for historical plaques.

Sent: Thursday, May 13, 2010

I slept horrible last night. We had big thunderstorms every two hours or so, lots and lots of rain. I think I was awake from 2:45–4:30 am. I am going to try to nap today. I don't want to look sickly for the awards ceremony tonight. I have to get up and shake hands with the mayor!

Talk to you soon, Love, Stacey

Sent: Thursday, May 20, 2010
Subject: Koby

What a little stinker and a smarty. Koby came home from a playdate and asked me to write my signature big on a piece of paper so he could see it. I complied. He secretly went into his bedroom with his backpack. I barged in a couple of minutes later to find him with a "RED" note from school trying to forge my signature. He claims he didn't do it. He has been having a little trouble since the sub started on the 23rd of April. Only a couple more weeks to go....

Stacey

Sent: Wednesday, June 23, 2010

Hi, Mom,

The kids had a good day at camp. I am debating about martial arts for them tonight. It is very sticky out, and a storm is approaching right now.

I had a good day. It was nice to sit for three plus hours. I was glad I brought snacks because I did not get out until 1:30. I met a woman there who flew from India to receive treatment in the U.S. She is driving 40 minutes to see my doctor because she likes him. I thought it was ironic that we have so many Indian doctors and a woman flew from Bombay to receive treatment here. She has no insurance, so it is all out of pocket. The sad thing is she has two young children in India, but she said they were using Skype to communicate.

I did quite a bit of clothing/garage sale organizing when I got home. I am taking a break now and preparing an easy dinner. Better go see when that big storm is going to hit.

Love Stacey

Sent: Wednesday, June 23, 2010
Subject: Superman

Hi, all,

Tommy got back from his bike trip today. They did a 60-mile ride yesterday and 20 or 30 the day before. Three months after heart surgery with no practice. Pretty cool. He is thinking of starting martial arts again next week. (He is still seeing a cardio PT, so they will continue to monitor.) His legs are a little sore tonight.

Time for sleep. I am on my last treatment in this round and doing fine so far.

Love Stacey

Sent: Wednesday, July 21, 2010
Subject: Re: hi

Hi, Mom,

Kassia is off to her scrapbook camp in a few minutes. Digging through pictures made me think about scrapbooking as my next big project. I have sooo many pictures.

Yesterday we went to martial arts class. It felt really good to work out. The instructor had me lead most of the class in doing forms. That felt good, too. I was relieved to remember most of them.

I did not do the sparring at the end of class, although I am wanting to do some non-contact sparring once I am a little more sure-footed. The neuropathy should subside over the next couple of months.

Last night we went to the outdoor concert at the park. It makes for an easy evening. We stop and get a $5 pizza to eat at the park. We bring our chairs and a blanket. The kids either watch the music or run around the park with their friends. Last night was especially nice because Tom got home in time to join us. Much of the music was from the '70s and '80s. The band was called Libido Funk Project. Interesting, eh?

I had a blood draw this a.m. Reds and whites were OK, had to get an injection for platelets, and I will need to get another tomorrow and a blood count on Friday. Feeling a bit like a pincushion lately, but I am thankful my energy has been adequate since Monday. I hate dragging the kids to these appointments, which should be a couple of minutes but wind up being an hour. They sat patiently today, so I rewarded them with donuts.

My garden is starting to produce cukes, zucchini, and eggplant. I see lots of stir fry in my future. That's the latest report from Elgin. What a nice summer day!

Love Stacey

Sent: Saturday, August 14, 2010
Subject: We made it

Hi Mom,

We arrived at Fay Lake about 2:30. The kids and Tom swam and went out in the boat. I took Midnight for a walk and relaxed.

I would say Fay Lake has gotten a little funkier. They have shored up a few of the cabins and probably saved them. There are three other people here. Our cabin is sufficiently clean, and the owners are nice.

It's nice and peaceful here.

Love Stacey

Sent: Sunday, August 15, 2010
Subject: Swimming

Koby started to doggie paddle yesterday. He said it was the pool and this place that made him do it. He is excited about swimming again. It is much cooler today.

Stacey

Sent: Monday, August 16, 2010
Subject: Hi

We are getting a motor for the boat here and going out later this a.m. The sun is out, but it is breezy and cool. The kids swam yesterday evening in spite of low 60 temps. I think there will be swimming action today. Koby is actually swimming now and is very excited. He said he will always remember this place because he learned to swim here. We are having a good time.

Love Stacey

Sent: Friday, September 03, 2010
Subject: our little whippersnapper

Hello,

Seven days into the school year, and I was greeted by Koby's teacher after school. Apparently, he had a bad afternoon. Fingers crossed we won't have a repeat. He did not get to play with his friends or play the computer. He was oozing with sweetness when we got home, though. He was helpful and also painted me a wonderful flower picture.

I did not have to get a shot today. I am glad because I am still a little punky since the shot on Wednesday. I am going to rest for about 30 minutes and decide whether I want to do the black belt class at 5:30. I am thinking it is not going to happen because we have some running around for birthday presents beforehand. I did not realize the sleepover was a birthday party. Somehow, I missed that. I hope you are having a good day.

Love Stacey

Sent: Monday, September 06, 2010
Subject: weekend

Hi, Mom,

On Sunday, we had a cookout. As we were finishing up, neighbor friends came by on their bikes. They stopped by to have a beer with us which for some led to another and another.... Soon a couple of other neighbors joined in. The kids and dogs played and played. We visited and had some laughs.

Today we did the bike ride. We went along the river to Walton Island and fed the ducks. It was a nice ride. We caught a few sprinkles coming back and then went to Dairy Queen. Tonight, I made vegetable soup with several garden veggies. I was surprised to find it was a hit with everyone. Talk to you soon.

Love Stacey

Sent: Monday, September 13, 2010
Subject: today

Hi, Mom,

What a nice day! I got out a little (walked with Midnight, walked to school) but mostly did inside stuff. I think I was on the phone for a good part of the morning re-arranging appointments, etc.

I saw my oncologist today. Everything looked good. My temp was 99.3, but I just got done driving around in a hot car, in traffic, running on fumes. I did get to talk to him about the potential for surgery, and it looks like they are leaning towards it. He said I was doing "very well" and that things seemed under control for now—thus, they were comfortable with a brief break in the chemo. I should know on Monday about the findings and recommendations. Hope to spend some of the morning in the yard.

Love Stacey

Stacey underwent surgery at this time to remove the diseased area of her colon.

Sent: Wednesday, October 13, 2010
Subject: doctor today

Hi, Mom,

I saw my doctor today. My bloodwork was improving—still a little anemic. I'll have to invest in that iron skillet or start loving steaks, I guess. I will start chemo again on the 27th without Avastin. Avastin will be added a couple weeks after that. I'll also have another CT scan once the healing has progressed.

Feeling better today. Still somewhat tired, and my nose is a little runny... a little cold perhaps? I may pick up around here a little. Other than that, I will take it easy.

Love Stacey

A special surprise for the kids was planned for Christmas 2010. Instead of the usual Christmas presents under the tree on Christmas morning, the family was going to Costa Rica!

Sent: Wednesday, October 20, 2010
Subject: hi

Hi, Mom,

It is a beautiful day here. I have been very lazy this morning. I did get out and do some shopping. I picked up a package of tulip bulbs and some yard bags. I guess that means I should get outside and enjoy some yardwork.

We have been busy running around trying to get passports the last couple of days now that tickets for the secret trip have been purchased. I am happy I bought tickets when I did even though the flight plan is screwy. I looked this morning, and the flights had nearly doubled in cost.

We had an interesting afternoon yesterday trying to keep this thing a secret.

First of all, I had to drag the kids to Walgreens to get their passport photos. "How come we have to get our pictures taken?" Me: "We are getting passports in case we ever want to take you to Canada." That was not too hard to get through, but it did arouse some suspicion, I am sure.

Next, we had to turn in the passport applications for the kids. Both parents had to be present with the kids, so Tom had to take off work early. The Elgin office was all booked up, so we had to drive to Geneva—15 miles away. I am sure our jumping through hoops to get down to that office on that day seemed a little strange to the kids.

When we arrived at the office and went up to the counter, I explained to the woman that our trip and destination was a surprise and she vowed to secrecy. The kids were hanging out behind me in line as the woman carefully went through our paperwork.

A few minutes later, I turned around and who did I see but my oncologist? He is such a sweet man. He greeted me with a big hug and then asked what we were doing at the Kane County courthouse. I said we were getting passports. Naturally he was interested and asked where and when we were going (even though I had told him at a previous appointment, and he gave me his blessing to take the trip). The kids were now all looking at us, and I chuckled and told him it was a surprise for the kids, and I would tell him another time. He was a little embarrassed for having caused a potential breach.

After the kids' applications were complete, the woman gathered papers and the photos for Tom's renewal. Here we ran into several glitches. First, was the ancient copy of his birth certificate—I remarked that he was just very old. They decided it may be passable, or they may send it back demanding another copy. Secondly, there was a problem with his photo.

The woman got out her plastic template and revealed that his head was too big (hee hee). At this time, it was decided that we would have to wait to fulfill his application. The woman and I started to calculate the number of weeks we had before the trip to make sure it could all be done in time. Another woman behind the counter was brought into the fray. She was not aware of my secret pact with the first woman and practically shouted out, "So are you leaving before or after Christmas?" By now the kids are wide-eyed and looking very interested. Tom asked them to take a seat on the other side of the room where they whispered back and forth—no doubt speculating on what we were up to.

We left the office with our applications 90% complete. Tom would have to have his photo re-taken and would have to find another post office or courthouse to go to for finalization. On the ride home, the car was very silent. Tom and I wondered if we should just let the "cat out of the bag" at this point but chose not to because an empty-handed Santa is going to look very bad. Instead I said our family needs a "Don't Ask Don't Tell" policy on this topic.

The real test is when I am going to have to take the kids into the travel doctor to get a typhoid shot. Dragging them in for photos and paperwork is one thing, but when I tell them they need to get a shot, there is going to have to be an explanation.

I am waiting to hear back to get the OK on a typhoid shot from my oncologist. I would have asked him yesterday but decided to respect him on his day off. I am sure he runs into patients everywhere. I may not need the shot because I had one just over five years ago.

Love Stacey

Sent: Thursday, October 28, 2010
Subject: hello

Hello,

I am feeling good today after a good night's sleep. I sleep like a kitten with this chemo. That is a really good thing.

I am a little overwhelmed with getting behind on things and the flurry of activities Halloween brings. I want it to be fun! I surprised the kids and decorated the front porch on my super-energetic day while they were at school. It is really cool. We still have to finalize the costumes, so there is some shopping to do.

The other things to do beside Halloween shopping are: overdue library books, a bag full of mail to go through and bills to pay, plan dinner, do laundry, walk the dog (optional), the kids need to go to Kyuki-do this week, dance class tomorrow.... Yikes! I need to get off the computer. I go to the doctor at 11:30 today. I am sure I will be there until the kids get out of school. I won't feel like doing much this afternoon or evening, especially driving. How to get it all done? I just need to prioritize, starting with overdue bills and phone calls first. If I organize my bags, I can do some from the doctor, but I am REALLY enjoying that Barbara Kingsolver book, and it is nice to leave everything behind and just sit and read while I am there.

I did yoga last night and was the only one there besides one other woman and the teacher. We spent the first half of class talking. The one woman is an eight-year survivor of two different cancers and was given eight months to live when she was diagnosed at 45. She is now 53. She has been through the same treatment as me. She is working, very active, and looks great. Her attitude and actions sounded similar to mine. She gave me her phone numbers. I think she will be a good resource and possibly friend. It was nice to get back to yoga. It was an easy restorative class with some meditation.

My oncologist came by and said hi yesterday while I was there. He was raving about how well the surgery and recovery went. He thought we really proved Dr. A. wrong, who was skeptical going into it. I have to applaud Dr. A. for a very good job, though. Coffee is done. Time to hop into action here.

Love Stacey

Sent: Wednesday, November 03, 2010
Subject: hi

Hi, Mom,

It's turning out to be a nice afternoon here after a rainy gray morning. So, you were not happy with the election results either? It was a mixed bag here locally with some very tight races.

Saw my doc this a.m. for blood counts. I am thrilled I did not have to get a shot. Platelets were low at 83, but I will be checked on Monday to see if they climb back over 100 on their own. I talked to him about the trip and got his complete blessing on anything I want to do if I am up for it. Ziplining and a three-hour easy hike at around 3,000–5,000-foot altitude are on the list, so I better keep my strength up. The last couple of days involve beach and poolside, so that will be good. Of course, I will allow myself a siesta every day.

He said they will alter my treatment schedule if needed as it gets closer, so I do not get "hit" while traveling. I am also having a scan on Tuesday. That will be interesting as it has been four months, two of which I was not being treated. Looking forward to yoga tonight. My house is a mess—yikes!

Stacey

Sent: Monday, November 08, 2010
Subject: Re: awesome day

It was a good day here. I felt a little crummy this weekend from the Neulasta shot and was sore from yoga. I took it real easy and feel great today. The doc may adjust future shots, or we hope my counts won't dive bomb as much without the oxaliplatin drug, which I am done with. The counts rebounded nicely this time.

Don't worry about not being here for the scan. It is really quick and easy. Last time, I was in and out in ten minutes. It was performed fully dressed, lay down, dye injected, a couple of pictures—done. The results will probably be in by Friday.

Kassia got straight A's, and Koby's teacher said, "Koby is an ideal student." Aleks got his report card last week and had all A's and two B's. (ISAT score 99% nationally again in math, but that was one subject he got a B in—go figure). Not a bad first quarter. Proud mama.

Gotta get these kids in bed by 8 p.m. This time change screws them all up.

Love Stacey

Sent: Wednesday, November 10, 2010
Subject: Hi

Hi, Mom,

I sent you a message about my CT scan. I am happy with the results.

The doc is also changing my treatment so I will not have to come in on Thursdays. I will still have the pump Wednesday–Friday. He said it may help with my counts.

I guess I can look forward to a platelet shot this week. My counts were below threshold today, and they are going ahead with treatment.

I am sitting here waiting to get started. We are very far behind today. I think I will need to call my friends to pick up the kids. I'm glad I brought plenty of snacks. I will call you soon!

Love Stacey

Sent: Wednesday, November 17, 2010
Subject: Re: hello

Mmmmm pie!

It will be great to see everyone for Thanksgiving, especially since our visit could be short.

I think the kids' wheels are really turning about hints of this trip. Aleks was telling me about a classmate whose family is going to Greece, Egypt, and Spain over Thanksgiving. He sounded a bit jealous.

There was also a huge surge of interest in learning Spanish this weekend. The kids had Spanish books out and were practicing up. Hmmmmm....

Yesterday Koby said he wanted to go on another trip like Seattle on an airplane.

I didn't get my house clean today. I got the yardwork done, a load of dishes and a load of laundry—and a long dog walk. Oh well, a little each day. Time to get the kids.

Love Stacey

Hi, Mom,

Yippity, skippity, my blood counts were fine today, so no shots. They doctor also suggested we skip next week because of the holiday complication. It was his idea, not mine, but that was what I was hoping for. I am feeling very good and energetic today, so I imagine next week will be even better especially without the shots. Look out because I will have a big appetite on Thursday.

Love Stacey

Sent: Saturday, December 04, 2010
Subject: Re: snow

We got some snow, probably 3–4 inches. It was nice wet snow, and the kids have been playing in it most of the day. It is pretty. I got a wreath the other day, and the kids and Tommy may get a tree this afternoon. They are talking about chopping one down. I might take it easy because I'm tired. I had a mammogram an hour ago and got a little lightheaded from that. Maybe I was holding my breath, or it was creeping me out.

Last night I took the kids to the black belt class. Afterwards there was a potluck with lots of yummy homemade Mexican food. I brought a couscous salad, which was good, but it didn't quite go with the theme.

Tomorrow is decorating day at church. I am not sure if we will go or not. The snow makes it feel so much more like Christmas. We will be decorating the house for sure.

Maybe I will start a soup for dinner. It has been a nice lazy day.

I hope Grandma feels better. It is nice you are so close and can check on her.

Happy decorating!

Love Stacey

CHAPTER 20
A Return to Costa Rica

Sent: Monday, December 13, 2010

I only have four days (without kids) to do my top-secret packing and printing out our reservation confirmations and such. That is the fun stuff! I'll clean a little this morning for the party, and then I'll start the packing.

I go in for a blood test this afternoon at 1:40. I am hoping counts are good so I can have the treatment on Wednesday. There isn't much wiggle room with this trip coming up.

Hope you have a good day and that Grandma's consultation goes well. Say hi to her. I need to drop her an e-mail soon.

Love Stacey

Sent: Monday, December 13, 2010
Subject: today

Well, Kassia had the perfect little party. She planned the activities and the sequencing of everything, and it went very smoothly with just enough time for everything. She has a great group of friends.

They all work together so nicely.

I did not have to get a shot today. I was pleased my white count was in the normal range, and my platelets were up to 97 from 70. My red count has been hanging around 10.5. My doctor did not seem as impressed as I was. He said, "Eh, you are borderline (for platelets), but I think you will be OK for Wednesday." Oh well. I was happy to get in and out of there quickly today. In the last 2.5 months, I have only had one shot for my blood, and I don't think that one was necessary.

I think the party girl is in her room trying on some new makeup. She got a little kit from Stella.

Talk to you soon.

Love Stacey

Sent: Saturday, December 18, 2010 8:48 PM
Subject: hi

Hi, Mom,

I think I have the kids packed. I also have my clothes picked out and ironed in a pile. It is good to have that done. There are so many other little details to work out. I bought first aid stuff today. For an active vacation with three kids, you must have a little kit with all of those boo-boo essentials.

I will really miss coming to Boscobel for Christmas. You guys have a way of making the holidays extra special. I think it was a wise choice, though. Tommy keeps having little things pop up at work, and I am trying to stay calm, and sane, and keep my energy up.

We will probably go to church on Christmas Eve. We usually have a nice service with candles and carols. Christmas morning will be the big reveal. The only awkward thing is the kids won't have much to play with. Robin is coming over around noon. Tommy might make his pierogi dinner again.

I was not feeling so good today. I am sure I am fighting one of these bugs that are going around again. It doesn't feel like it is going to turn into anything big—just tired, cold, and a little achy. I just hope it isn't drawn out for a few days. I was careful today and cut out all the martial arts stuff I had planned to do. Koby tested for his brown stripe today. Tom took him, and I took a little nap. I was happy he had all 36 moves of his form memorized this time.

Love Stacey

Sent: Tuesday, December 21, 2010
Subject: Re: snow

We had the perfect kick-off to holiday break with the snowstorm yesterday evening. I think we got about four inches. The kids have been playing in it.

We just did our martial arts class, and now the kids are eating lunch. Koby is upset because he thinks Aleks got more milk than him and now the milk is gone. I want to take them rock climbing at the Centre this afternoon because Kassia has never done it. I think it would be good practice to get strapped onto ropes and climb high. :) Kassia really wants to do it. I am having second thoughts because it looks like we have a little too much drama here. Well, I better go. Enjoy your snow! Stacey

Sent: Tuesday, December 21, 2010
Subject: hi again

Hi, Mom,

So, we made it to the rock climbing. Koby's only fear was, "Does my butt look big?" He was worried that the straps squished his butt and made it look big. Well, that (chunky, LOL) 60-pounder scaled up that 35-foot rock tower with ease. Neither Kassia or Aleks went to the top this time. I will say that Kassia did 100 feet. About 10 feet up and then back down about 10 times. She said it was because she liked the ride down and not that she was afraid to go up high. I think she went up 20 feet one of the times.

I am getting down to the wire on things.... We have a busy activity-filled day tomorrow. I have my blood check, and I am scheduled to see Dr. Jaena again in the morning. In the afternoon, we have plans to meet up with friends for sledding.

I'm not sure whether Tommy has to work on Friday or not. He had a meeting yesterday, and it did not sound like they were treating it as a holiday. Christmas is one of their listed paid holidays, so they should get a day either Friday or Monday. He enjoyed the meeting because they mentioned a scenario where he would become a VP sometime down the road.

Time to start dinner. I am thinking chicken and sweet potatoes and black beans.

Love Stacey

Sent: Wednesday, December 22, 2010

Had good doctor visits this a.m. No shots. I went on to see Dr. Jaena, though, and had more acupuncture. She was feeling some good vibes, and I checked out with very good energy. Must be the trip excitement. Tommy has been upping my green juice, too. I've felt very energetic the last couple of days.

Took the kids sledding with Janet. It was fun but also interesting. A man confronted us about a sled that belonged to one of his kids and acted like he wanted to fight about it in front of all the kids. He was EXTREMELY out of line. All I could really do was laugh, which probably made him madder. Towards the end, I was ready to play black belt and knock him on his butt. He got very close to Janet and said, "At least your kids seem better behaved than you!" He was acting like he was in a bar and wanted to take it "out to the parking lot," and she really did nothing to provoke it.

Time to make some burritos for dinner. I am planning a quiet night in front of the TV and laptop.

Love Stacey

Sent: Thursday, December 23, 2010
Subject: hi

Hi, Mom,

Well, our plans are coming along, and things are falling into place. Tomorrow is cleaning day. On Saturday, we will fine-tune the packing.

Kassia made another cake to bring to Grandma Carole and Grandpa Gary's.

I almost messed up in front of the kids last night. That puts Tommy and I 1:1. He did not think the kids really noticed. We will give you a call on Saturday. I cannot believe that tomorrow is Christmas Eve.

Stacey

Sent: Saturday, December 25
Subject: Merry Christmas

Hi, Mom,

Merry Christmas to you!

Well, the secret is out… each of the kids had a different reaction. It was all good.

I came downstairs at 5:44 when I was sure I heard someone walking around. I was met by Aleks, who had already been through the suitcase and stocking and had everything carefully sorted. He was excited and had a smile on his face. I did not expect squeals and jumping.

Kassia was the next one up and was still waking up when she came out and Aleks told her, "We are going to Costa Rica."

Her first response was, "Why?" and she said, "I thought we were going to Grandma and Grandpa's—but I made a cake." She was confused and did not know where the trick ended. She thought we were teasing her about the trip, and she expected to find another Santa gift tucked in her clothes. She also needed clarity on what was from Santa and what was from us.

Koby was the last one up. He was just happy-go-lucky about everything. When Aleks said we are going to Costa Rica tomorrow, he asked, "That's farther than Wisconsin, right? Is it in Africa?" We did figure out that it isn't much farther away than Seattle.

He has since then asked the cutest questions.

"Do they eat shrimp there? Maybe I will try shrimp."

"I think it will be kind of Hanukkah there because they don't have snow or Christmas trees...."

As far as who knew... Aleks said he kind of had it figured out. He even admitted to talking to Josh about it. "Don't get too excited, because I am not sure yet, but I think we are going to Costa Rica." What led him to figure it out?

1. When Tommy was on the phone and said, "I'm going to Cost..."

2. He saw me on the Travelocity website.

3. He saw me looking at scuba/snorkel gear.

Kassia and Koby had no idea.

I must say they LOVED the money, cameras, and wallets!

Well, Tommy went back to bed. I am just enjoying sitting here with the kids among the gift wrap fielding the occasional question. It is such a nice white Christmas, but it will be good to be transported out of winter. We will talk to you later.

Love Stacey

Sent: Monday, December 27, 2010
Subject: Ole

Hi, Buenos Dias,

We made it! Flights through el Salvador and Guatemala went very smoothly. Top-notch aircraft.

We had a nice room upgrade to a two-bedroom suite. Sweet!

It is very windy in San Jose. It is warming up this a.m. with clear skies.

Just had a wonderful breakfast with fresh papaya and pineapple.

Tommy and the kids just left to get the rental car. I will shower, put some sunscreen on, and lay by the pool. I may leave long sleeves on as it is still cool.

I feel great even after hauling luggage yesterday. The kids are being very good and so interested in everything. Off to the cloud forest this afternoon. Adios.

Love Stacey

Sent: Tuesday, December 28, 2010
Subject: Day two

Hello from sunny Costa Rica,

We made it to the Monteverde area yesterday. The last 15 miles were on roads similar to going out to Laurie and Todd's with some hairpin turns, slightly narrower gravel roads (with potholes), and towards the end, the drop-offs looked to be several thousand feet without guardrails. The scenery was beautiful, and we were greeted by the cloud forest with a big glowing rainbow.

It was very breezy and misty late yesterday. The night was cool. A bit cooler than normal, they say. We were happy the winds died down, and it was a pretty nice morning.

We went to the cloud forest reserve today for a fabulous 3.5-hour hike. We saw some new kinds of birds that I can't spell and a new kind of mammal that I can't spell. One of the birds was a mottled owl, and the other was a blue-crowned motmot. It was very interesting— we had an excellent guide.

Everyone was surprised at how well the kids behaved on the hike, and the guide gave us a discount because of their good behavior. We just took them out for a nice lunch at the Blue Morpho because we saved so much on the hike. The kids only ate half their subs, so it looks like an easy dinner tonight.

Now for some downtime, and then we might go out to the frog pond later, another popular attraction here. We will walk to town and buy a couple more groceries. We found the shopping a little cheaper than home but not much. The kids have used up their cameras and want to buy another one with some of their money.

I am going to go soak up a little of this sunshine and dry out from the morning hike.

I can tell I might be a little sore tomorrow after the long and sometimes uphill hike at 5,000 feet altitude. But I am feeling good. Ziplining tomorrow. :) Love, Stacey

Sent: Thursday, December 30, 2010
Subject: Hi

Hello,

We have had an active week so far. Ziplining was a blast. Tommy said it is the most fun he has had in a long time. After Monteverde, we traversed some crazy roads to get to Arenal.

So far, all is going according to plan.

The kids were enjoying birds and wildlife this a.m. Breakfasts are so good here with fresh fruit and local ingredients. We did another long hike this a.m.

The volcano erupted for the first time in four months. It was too foggy to see. Hopefully we will get a show before we go. We are heading to town to get pizza. Afterwards, we will do the pool and hot tub. Off to Jaco tomorrow—beach time! I feel very good! Pura vida! Stacey

Sent: Friday, December 31, 2010
Subject: Happy new year

We are in Jaco relaxing after a long day of driving. Started the day with a flat tire. We drove to town slowly as it was not completely flat. It was fixed in less than 30 minutes and cost 2,000 colones or four dollars.

It's a bit more urban here. I am already hearing firecrackers. It promises to be a loud night. The hotel is compact. The kids are enjoying the pool and trampoline outside of our room. Tommy and I can enjoy our porch while the kids are playing.

Tomorrow we go to Manuel Antonio Park for some nice beaches and possible monkey sightings.

It is very warm here and dry. A nice change. I am not sure how we will celebrate our anniversary tonight.

Love to all, Stacey

Saturday, January 01, 2011
Subject: Hi

We had a nice day at Manuel Antonio. The beach was beautiful, and we saw monkeys. A raccoon almost ran away with Kassia's cola.

Tommy and Aleks are watching the end of the Rose Bowl in the room. I'm watching the other kids swim.

Love Stacey

Sent: Sunday, January 02, 2011
Subject: On our way home

Well, I think we got plenty of sun over the last two days.

Today we relaxed and took a trip to shops and the beach. We just finished a nice pizza dinner. We will finish packing tonight. We will leave here between 6 and 7 a.m. It is 1.5 hours to the airport. Flight at 10:30. We will be in Guatemala until our 8:30 p.m. flight. Eight hours is a long time at an airport, but it is a nice one. They even have Sony PlayStations.

The kids are having their last swim. Tommy is enjoying a nice cerveza.

The kids have already decided that they don't want to go to school on Tuesday.

What an awesome trip. It is hard to see it end.

Love Stacey

CHAPTER 21
Treatments and Treating Oneself

Sent: Wednesday, January 05, 2011
Subject: Hi

Hi, Mom,

Just got weighed, and I've gained 5 lbs. 126 with shoes—I've always thought 130 would be a good weight. I don't know if it was the holidays or those hearty Costa Rican breakfasts. All I need now is Mom's Christmas cookies to top me off.

My blood counts were pretty good, except platelets were 96K, but I will get the full treatment anyway. I should be done here before 1 p.m.

The kids were anxious to get to school today. I promised to take their cameras in. I got my pictures developed... there were 353! I think I will sift through them before I subject anyone to a slideshow like that. I will work on that and my journal today while I am here maybe with some Bob Marley on the iPod to extend those vacation vibes. Have a great day!

Love Stacey

Sent: Tuesday, January 11, 2011
Subject: hello

Hi, Mom,

Midnight and I went on a long walk this afternoon. He really needed it as I have been slacking since the trip. It was a nice day for a walk with the fresh snow and warmer temps. I think I walked about two miles today.

It has been so much work getting caught up on things. I've accomplished a little each day. Finally, the trip laundry is done, but the regular laundry piles up.

I got a little design job today. I am going to help the neighbors with the bakery that I did with their basement. Instead of taking money, I may ask to put business cards in the bakery for advertising. We will see....

I am looking forward to our visit next weekend. It will be so nice to see everyone. I'm making cookies with Kassia. I have to go stick them in the oven.

Love Stacey

Sent: Monday, January 17, 2011
Subject: hi

Hello,

We had a nice snowy day here. It has turned to rain and sleet this evening.

I might not get my full treatment this week because the platelet counts were still too low, 84K. He may adjust the treatment in the future so they don't get knocked down as much. I will definitely get the Avastin on Wednesday. There would be a small chance they would rise above 90K by then, and I would get the full treatment. My CEA count held pretty steady this month and was at 3.7. I am still going to take that as a good sign.

I still have been feeling terrific! I mean really terrific. I hope it lasts and I don't get Aleks' cold. He is functioning but is now coughing and is pretty stuffed up.

I have to make a birthday cake tomorrow. We have a PTA fundraiser/McDonalds night tomorrow, so I guess that will be the birthday dinner. Maybe I will make Tommy something else extra special for dinner. I will talk to you soon. Looking forward to that Bears-Packers game.

Love Stacey

Sent: Tuesday, January 25, 2011
Subject: peas

Hi, Mom,

Well I made Kassia eat her peas last night and, apparently, she has a significant allergy to green peas, too. Her lips swelled a little, and her throat hurt. I gave her two teaspoons of Benadryl, and it cleared. Scary. I guess I should take her in and have her tested for all legumes. I did suspect that she has reacted to lentils, chick peas, and lima beans in the past. She seems fine with pinto beans and green beans. If she is that allergic to other legumes, she should probably be carrying medication at all times.

My busy day yesterday turned out a little easier than planned. My design appointment was postponed, and I was able to change my afternoon doctor's appointment so I could do it before the kids were home. Kassia and I were able to make four dozen cookies for the cookie-tasting contest today. It should be fun. What a good idea for a fundraiser.

My platelets were OK yesterday. It was the white count that was low. That was why I got the shot. Hopefully they will be good enough for treatment tomorrow.

I have a pretty quiet day today, but it will fill up if I go to martial arts and do a dog walk, which I plan to do.

Love Stacey

Thursday, January 27, 2011
Subject: Re: Today

Sounds like you have a busy day today! Maybe you will get this message between appointments. Say hi to Grandma for me.

Yes, they did change my treatment, only slightly. My doctor said they took the part out that probably has the most impact on the blood counts but least impact on the overall efficacy. I won't be getting any 5-FU during my Wednesday sessions. It will only be delivered in the take home pump. He will check my counts on Friday when I get the pump off to see if there is any downward trend starting. The strategy now is to avoid the shots as much as possible, but I did tell him I did not want to compromise the effectiveness of my treatment at this time.

I was tired last night, but I think I was still feeling the effect of Monday's shot. I did get to yoga class though. Today I am feeling fine. No nausea at all. I slept well and am not tired. I finished off the Costa Rican coffee and then had some spicy Indian food for lunch, so my stomach is fine....

The cookie bake-off went well. The turnout wasn't great, but it was fun for those who attended. The chili cook-off was more popular, and the upcoming tamale cook-off may be even better! I can't say I have ever cooked a tamale. I may challenge myself and perhaps surprise some people with some vegetarian tamales. I know I have some recipes in my cookbooks. I imagine some in our school have it down to an art, though. Kassia did not win with her eggless Toll House cookies. They were really good, and we enjoyed making them.

I think we got an inch of snow, and now it is slowing down. I have had a nice quiet morning with no appointments for a change. I scheduled some classes at the LivingWell Center (for people affected by cancer). I am excited. One of them is a two-session creative writing course by our former yoga teacher. I like her a lot, and she just finished up some writing courses out in California, so I think she will have a lot to share. The second class is a Look Good, Feel Better class on makeovers for cancer patients. Attendees get a free package of top-of-the-line makeup. I haven't lost my eyebrows yet, but I am in need of some new makeup (hee hee). It is on Valentine's Day so I can give myself a Valentine's Day makeover and have a little present and surprise my sweetie when he gets home. Finally, I scheduled a reiki session.

Right now, I need to get ready for an appointment with Master Kim to schedule our next "green" seminar, which I think will be February 26th. Have a great day! Love you, Stacey

Sent: Saturday, January 29, 2011
Subject: Re: Mother

Hi, Mom,

I was sorry to hear about Grandma but so thankful you and Gary were there for her. I did not get your e-mail until tonight. We were cleaning and organizing maniacs today, and I was not on the computer or Facebook at all. Let her know I am thinking about and praying for her.

At 3 p.m. Tommy took Koby and Trevor to Legoland. I think they had fun. I went to an open house at Simple Balance Holistic Center where Dr. Jaena is. I was surprised that one of the guest speakers was Wende, the former owner of our home. She gave me a free 30-minute reiki session (her new specialty). It was cool.

After that, I came home with some Little Caesar's pizzas. Koby opened his presents (Thank you! He was very happy). He got his wish of smashing his face in a cake. I got it on video and will send it soon. It sounds like you could use a laugh. Maybe you can show it to Grandma, too, if she is up to it. He did not look like he enjoyed it as much as he thought he would. Afterwards, we had an ice cream cake that he did not stick his face in.

He is having a sleepover with Trevor and has banned us all to the upstairs so that they can watch TV or eat whatever they want. I better check on them soon.

Tomorrow I am serving a big breakfast at 8 am. Kassia and Aleks have their black belt midterm at 10 a.m. That is a huge step in getting their black belts.

At 4 p.m. we are getting a family picture taken—finally. It will be just a cheap quickie at Sears. We will see how that goes. I'll be checking my e-mail on my phone for any updates about Grandma. Love Stacey

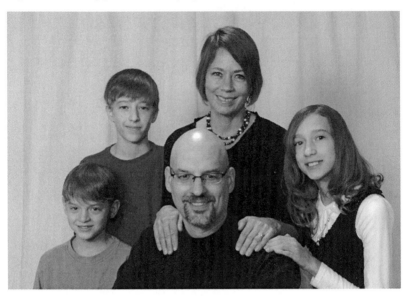

Sent: Thursday, February 03, 2011
Subject: today

Hi, Mom,

I hope things are looking up for Grandma, and she is looking forward to going home soon. I got the picture of her and the flowers. I thought she was looking good in the picture.

Things are slowly getting back to normal here. I got into my doctor's office. I was expecting chaos there with everyone changing appointments, but it was calm. There was a power outage there until this a.m., so no appointments yesterday. My bloodwork was great—some of the best numbers I have seen! Even my hemoglobin was above 12. So, lucky me—no shots, and I don't go back until Wednesday.

Tonight is the writing class. I look forward to that and think the roads should be fine for the 12-mile drive.

This just in... NO SCHOOL TOMORROW! That is three snow days in a row! Yikes. I think we will have to make a snowman tomorrow.

Love Stacey

Five Minute Writing Exercise
Feb. 3, 2011
By Stacey Reynolds

Cue Word: "Eyes"

I am standing with my mother in their Jamaica room—a room full of travel relics, dangling plants, and home to Sophie the cat!

It is a room full of life, a gathering place—a place where family meets to exchange stories and ideas—a place of love and laughter.

It is a room where my mother paints. She paints extraordinary portraits that capture the soul of the subject.

I have come to the room to view her latest creation, a portrait of my daughter, Kassia. I have seen this painting before on prior visits and watched it slowly coming to life.

It started as a black and white grayscale, but now that she has added the color, there is new life.

The painting leaves me with a warm feeling in my chest, for it reveals an innocence and beauty in my daughter that is very personal to me....

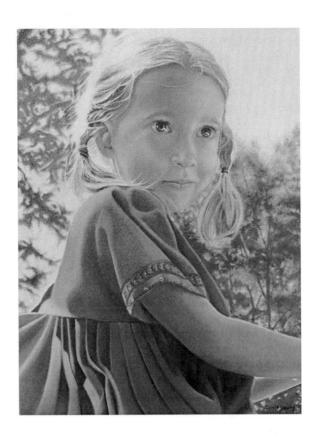

Sent: Wednesday, February 09, 2011
Subject: yucky day

Hi, Mom,

Well, it is one of those days when nothing is going right. First of all, it is minus 0 degrees. Secondly, I had to keep the boys home again. Mostly because Koby still had a fever yesterday. I think they are on the road to recovery (good news).

I went in for my treatment, and they warned me that there would be a wait because they were overbooked. They finally called me back, but I had to sit on a regular chair that is usually for visitors because the recliners were full. They were all backed up because of the snowstorm last week. They did my blood draw but found that my counts had dropped. Whites were only 2.8 (one of the lower readings I have had), and platelets were 73K. I should have had them double-check to make sure they were my counts. The name was handwritten instead of the usual computer printout, and they were very busy.

Anyway, I spoke to the doctor who was available, and he was unwilling to do any treatment, which is what I expected. He expects the counts to go up on their own, so I did not get shots. I am going to go in Friday voluntarily for a blood draw to see that they are indeed climbing again. The nurses said to do it Monday, but I want to make sure they are climbing by Friday. If I wait until Monday, there might not be anything they can do to raise them by my next treatment, which is scheduled for Wednesday. It seems my counts are dropping after 1.5 weeks instead of the usual five days. This might be important to note when designing my future treatments

While I was disappointed about the day, it might be a good thing anyway. I started to feel a little punky while I was sitting there, cold and a little bit of a dry cough. I feel like I am getting a cold. I did not have a fever when they took my temp. I need to stay in and stay warm, keep my reserves up, and probably stay away from sick people—ha! Like that is possible around here! I do feel better now that I am warming up in my bedroom. I may go down later and cook some leeks for soup.

Sorry to burden you with all of this stuff. You will be able to go out and get a medical degree after dealing with Grandma and me! I hope you are finding some time for yourself to catch up on a few things this week.

I am looking forward to reading and writing and resting this afternoon. I have the perfect excuse not to go out anywhere. I may even skip yoga this evening.

That's all for now. Tomorrow I should have all the kids back in school for the first time in 1.5 weeks! I should probably run out to the mall and pick up our family pictures. They have been ready since late last week. I will keep you posted. I love you! Stacey

Sent: Monday, February 14, 2011
Subject: Re: today

Hi, Mom,

It was a quiet day here. I got some laundry and housework done and waited on my sick boy. He ran a fever all day and slept a lot but did not seem uncomfortable or miserable. He was eating and drinking. I made some fresh-squeezed juice for him. He will not be able to go to school tomorrow because of the continuing fever. I will have to talk to his teacher because he has missed so much this month.

I did not get to go to my doctor's appointment. I don't think it will make much difference. The main reason they wanted me to come in was in case the platelets continued to go down.

I need a break! I have cancelled so many things so far this month. Mostly because I wasn't feeling good last week but also the kids (my make-up class, a reiki session, my writing class, Kyuki-do, yoga class... all the things that usually help me feel good). Tonight, I was trying to throw together a dinner and make cookies for Aleks' class for his birthday, and I burned the last pan of cookies. They had to go out to the store and buy some extras.

We had a really quick party for Aleks last night because Tommy did not get home until after 7. Everyone was so hungry and tired. Aleks liked his hat and appreciated the money. Valentine's Day today was equally chaotic.

I might reactivate my helper list. Things were moving along so well, and I was able to do so much, but it doesn't take long for things to get difficult. Midnight hasn't had a walk in a week now.

I was able to get a few healthy things to eat. You know it is bad when it feels like a nice break to get out to the grocery store!

I know by the end of the week we will be out of this mess, (well, some of it anyway). I am looking forward to those 50-degree temperatures, a nice walk in the sunshine, cracking the windows open a little. This too shall pass.

I am glad Grandma is getting settled in. I will let you know how tomorrow goes. The plan is to stay home with Koby. The afternoon gets crazy because both Kassia and Aleks have a Battle of the Books meet. Their schools compete against each other, and it is the last meet, so I really want to go. I am hoping Koby feels good enough by 3 p.m. to go with. At 7 p.m. we have a choral concert to attend for Aleks' school. I think I better take up meditation or medical marijuana or something! Eeeeks! Stacey

Sent: Tuesday, February 15, 2011
Subject: today

Hi, Mom,

I got Koby back in school today. He made it through the day. I won't hold my breath. I don't think he or Aleks are 100% yet.

I feel much better. I got a short dog walk in and went to martial arts. I still need to work to get my strength back up, but it felt good to get out and get moving!

We made it to the BOB meet. Aleks' school won, and Kassia's took second. It was fun to watch them compete. We were unable to go to the choral concert because Aleks was not feeling great tonight. I also found out it is very uncool for sixth-graders to go. I explained that his music teacher works hard....

I got my house clean because Minister Dan came over this morning. It was good to talk to him. It's nice that he is so close.

I will let you know how tomorrow goes. How was Grandma's appointment? Love, Stacey

On February 27, Stacey's maternal grandmother and Carole's mother, Lois Goldsmith, died at the age of 94. She had been diagnosed with leukemia six months before.

Sent: Thu, March 3, 2011 8:20
Subject: visitation

The family meets a little after three at the funeral home on Friday night. I don't know if everyone knew that or not. That might not be possible for some coming from far away, but whoever is there at that time, that is what we are supposed to do.

Carole/Mom

Sent: Thursday, March 03, 2011
Subject: Re: visitation

The Reynolds/Lesiewicz family will have to come in two shifts.

Stacey and kids will leave Elgin at 2 p.m., arriving in Boscobel for the visitation at around 6 p.m.

Tommy and Midnight will leave Elgin at around 6 or 6:30 and should be to Boscobel around 10 p.m. We plan to stay at your house and have a big family slumby in the "peach" room.

I am feeling energetic today. It gets crazy around here starting at 2:30. I am resting for the next two hours in anticipation of a big evening. Tomorrow morning, I just have a doctor's appointment and then have to go to the church for something. I hope to be all packed by then so I can rest before picking up the kids and heading out. Hope all is well there. I look forward to seeing you again.

Love Stacey

Sent: Wednesday, March 09, 2011
Subject: today

Hi, Mom,

Blood counts were good today.

I had a good talk with my doctor. Most of it was much of what I thought or what he has already told me. He said things could be stable for a month or for years—there is just no telling. He said that the medicines are working really well these days and that info on the internet is dated—also younger, active people fare better, and it depends on individual immune responses. There are other drugs available, if I progress, that they haven't used yet.

He has reduced medicines already and may even reduce to just Avastin if things continue to go well or if my bone marrow needs a break.

He did not think surgery was the next logical step, but that radio ablation radiation might be. (He said they did not think this was possible when he started with me, but we are getting closer—the PET scan will reveal how close we are.) He remains positive about all possibilities.

I am very comfortable with his judgment and think that he is knowledgeable (practicing over 30 years!), and he is constantly looking out for my best interest. I am lucky to have him for a doctor.

Stacey

Sent: Sunday, March 20, 2011
Subject: hello

Hi, Mom,

I felt pretty good yesterday after feeling poopy on Thursday and Friday. I was raking and digging like crazy yesterday. I got the corner with the signpost cleaned up. It took four lawn bags for that small area. There were all kinds of green things popping up underneath.

I also helped my neighbor with her basement colors yesterday. She was very happy with what I came up with.

The kids have their last martial arts mid-term today. They have to break a board. We are all getting excited. I think Tommy is taking them. I am going to church. It is Music Sunday, and we have a farmers market afterwards. I need to go to deliver my raspberry bushes. I dug them up and had multiple people wanting them. They were monsters, and I feared they would take over the yard. I am glad I found a home for them.

Burial at sea in progress for our recently departed fish "Cats." They were able to play "Taps" on the iPod as they flushed. We had him for about a week. Koby was pretty upset about it. I knew it was a bad idea.... Now the big decision... do we get another one? Or maybe he needs a turtle!

We better get ready to go. Maybe I will call later. Have a nice day!

Stacey

Sent: Monday, May 02, 2011
Subject: hi

Hi, Mom and Gary,

How about those Navy Seals? It is a good day for the U.S. of A.

Beautiful day here. I have a reiki appointment down at LivingWell at 11:00. I am looking forward to that. I may also get in to see the doctor for a platelet check and to see what he thinks about my sore back. He will probably say to go easy on those judo rolls!

Tonight, we have an open house at the middle school Aleks will go to. Can you believe it?

Tomorrow I may take the train into the city to meet up with Beth. We will go to some galleries in Bucktown and then out to lunch.

Thursday is Cinco de Mayo, and the school is having a festival again. Kassia is going to be one of the dancers this year. I am looking forward to all that good food. I hope that the weather stays nice.

I am sure I will be outside doing something today after my appointments.

Stacey

Sent: Thursday, May 12, 2011
Subject: Re: hot

Love the pictures! I sure enjoyed your visit. It was a very special Mother's Day. Thank you for bringing the truckload and also the picture. You know how dear that picture is to my heart. :) Now I need to get the wall painted to do it justice.

I have been gardening, too. I got some work done on the south side of the house on Tuesday. I did a little yesterday at 6:30 a.m. I found that a nice time to be out. Today I tackled the side garden but found that one wheelbarrow of weeds was about all I could do (hee hee, quite a bit actually). I did not want to overdo it. I have such a big, wonderful, and overwhelming garden! That wheelbarrow is very useful.

Love you, Stacey

CHAPTER 22

I'm Really Not Afraid of Anything Anymore

Sent: Monday, June 20, 2011

Hope you have an uneventful trip so far. It is cool and overcast at Fay Lake.

Jakoby is sick today. Hopefully he will revive by the afternoon, so he will be up for a boat ride. I think he managed to get a lot in between 3 and 10 p.m. yesterday... turtles, snails, catfish, frogs, swimming pool, rowboat, exercise machines, and S'mores.

We had a nice visit with Jon and Lesley. We grilled out and then watched the kids swim in the rain.

I started writing a long story today. It might even be a book. The setting will be very familiar to most of you. One of us will be sitting with Jakoby until he feels better. I don't mind the quiet time.

Hope the rain holds off today. I don't mind cool but could do without wet.

Stacey

This is the story Stacey wrote while on a family vacation at Fay Lake in June 2011. Not sure of a future with her family, she created one, projecting fourteen years into the future. The children are grown, and they gather once again at Fay Lake.

I am looking out a tiny window in a northeasterly direction. The storm is coming from the west, so I cannot see the darkness of the clouds that are about to move in. The lake and sky have a greenish cast. Quite opposite of the crimson sunset we enjoyed last night. My portable information device is charging on the table. I don't pick it up. Not to look at the radar, not to call. The storm is coming, and it looks like I will be riding it out alone in this tiny cabin. It makes no difference. *I am really not afraid of anything anymore.*

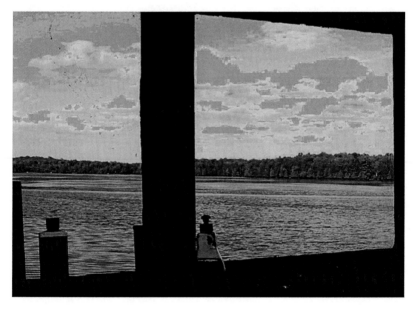

• • •

It has been fourteen years since we have been to Fay Lake. As always, it is in another stage of funky metamorphosis, which has always been a charm. Tom and I last brought the kids here in 2013. At that point, it was clear the economy, weather, and time itself, were taking a final toll on the little cabins. Gas prices had been over $5 a gallon all year, all but stopping the pipeline of Illinois tourists to the Northwoods. The rains had been unusually heavy for two summers, damping vacation spirits and contributing to more peeling shingles, paint, and the general sinking or sagging of the cabins over the water.

Finally, the tiny cabins and the owner's modest income could take no more. The resort closed after the summer season in '16. There was a post on the resort's Facebook page followed by 363 comments, all expressing deep regret and sharing fond memories. I had a strange feeling this place was going to live on, if not physically, in the hearts and photo albums of many.

The resort did live on. The economic climate in northern Wisconsin did improve primarily due to the high-speed rail that ran from the Chicago area on up the state as far as Wausau. Thanks to the power of the people, a very unpopular governor was removed from office. It took a couple of years for the new governor to undo the damage, but for the most part Wisconsin seems to be back on its progressive path, the rail project just being one of the projects that were renewed.

A businessman from some new pharmaceutical company based in Elk Grove Village purchased the Fay Lake Resort. He was able to scoop up a pretty good deal on the place and was ready to implement his big plans, at least until the fire came.

Three and a half years of extremely dry weather followed the wet summer in the Nicolet National Forest. The trees, once lichen covered, were now parched. The lake had gone down, too, and the docks were receding from the water like the gums of an old man who soon would need dentures. Apparently, the fire started at a campsite just east of Antigo. The winds had been blowing up to 30 mph that day, and the fire had all the fuel it needed to turn into a monster. A huge swath of the Nicolet was decimated. Tragically, this included part of the Menominee Indian reservation and its beautiful forest. Currently this area is in a state of renewal. Many hearts poured out to the people on the reservation. The governor put together a public works project that brought the people of Northern Wisconsin together to restore the lives of the Native Americans and its sustainable forest industry. Many people were employed in the process. Seeing the success of the program here, other states followed suit. Arizona implemented a program after wildfires there claimed 400,000 acres near the Lazy Creek reservation. We are seeing this kind of thing happen all over the country now especially with the freakishly common natural disasters that are occurring everywhere.

The fire touched the south end of Fay Lake, scorching the hillside behind the resort and engulfing cabins 5–10. The bar and house were also a total loss. The fire ended here. Some slow-moving thunderstorms pounded the area and assisted with the fire control, which now involved firefighters from four different states. The resort would sit for years before insurance funds could be processed and new plans could be drawn up.

It was a postcard that brought us up here again. We had received a few Fay Lake postcards in the past usually as the resort was passed from one owner to the next. I liked the look of the new cabins on the postcard. They were brightly colored and surrounded with wildflowers: spiderwort, Indian paintbrush, and Shasta daisies, to name a few. The card mentioned the cabins were "green" to minimize impact on the lake and to not further stress the area's water supply. I scanned my portable information device and found the new owner had worked very closely with the DNR and EPA to come up with a deal to build these zero-impact cabins over the lake again. The solution seemed brilliant to me, and I was convinced we had to go back. There was always something special about that place.

It was easy for me to find time to take a week and head north. I have been painting a lot lately. I am so fortunate to be able to stop and take a break now and then. The deadline for my latest commission does not come until August 19. I have over two months to fulfill that one. The gardens will wait for me, too. There are so many hands involved now that I really just sit back and enjoy their harvest.

I am also happy to say it has been a little easier to peel Tom away from his work these days. He is entering a stage of semi-retirement. I was so happy when my painting took off and my income from the paintings and gallery at the Center began dribbling in. Tom even took a few years off work on our solar business, which has had some very good times and allowed us to set aside what we need to retire and help fund the kids' college. Five years ago, he got back into the tech business and partnered with a younger coworker to form a new IT consulting firm. The business rode the wave of the improved economic climate that came with the president's re-election. Tom and his partner have been blessed with some really good staff, and he finally feels he can release himself from the stresses of the daily grind and take off. He's put more miles on his new Harley this year than he put on the previous one in five, and he's even grown some facial hair to go with it.

We took a train into Union Station and headed up to Wausau. It is a very pleasant three-hour ride. I especially enjoy the scenery north of Madison. The train speeds along I-39 between bluffs and over some beautiful bridges on the Wisconsin River. The food on the train wasn't bad either. There are three restaurant choices that cater there. One is your basic diner fare, which is served up in a really fun diner car. The design in the car is full of shiny stainless-steel surfaces embellished with plastic laminate. They even brought in an antique jukebox. The second car has a Wisconsin theme. I am not sure you can really get a meal, but if you like anything deep fried or on a stick, you can find it. You can also have your cheese any way you like it. I have always been a sucker for those deep-fried cheese curds, although I decided to pass this time. Last, but not least, there is ice cream. I came back for my favorite, "elephant tracks" cone, after finishing my meal at The Oasis. This car features ethnic fare, mostly Mediterranean, all made with fresh Madison area ingredients where possible. I found their falafel a little squishy for my taste, but the pita and the fresh ingredients were exquisite.

Tom was joining me for the first three days of the trip and then will be heading back to Chicago for his annual three-day bike trip. He has a group he has been getting together with for years. They are an unlikely bunch of Harley owners, but all seem to be joined at the hip with their bikes. He enjoys the company of these guys. They are a good group, full of intelligence and wit. I am happy Tom has found some comrades outside of work he likes to spend time with.

Once we get to Wausau, we will pick up a car at the U-Drive. We travel so much lighter these days. I have fond memories of our trips to Fay Lake with the kids: our Volvo wagon packed to the brim with its failing suspension sagging in the back. We always found a way to get it all in. With the cargo box on top, there was even room for Midnight, our four-legged friend. He was always there to share our Fay Lake adventures.

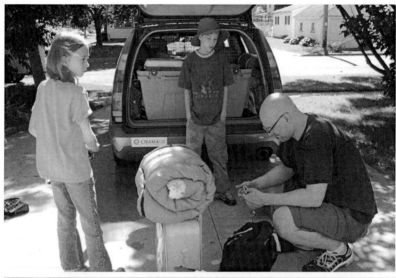

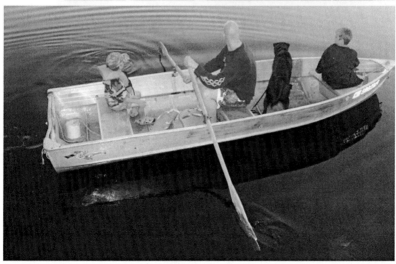

When we arrived at the lake, there was just a hint of familiarity. The winding road to the cabins looked the same. We almost missed the turn coming into the resort from Highway 139 simply because the sign was so hard to see as the sunlight was fading, and, somehow, we had lost our GPS signal outside of Crandon. I was glad to see the resort had not upgraded the signage. The old faded signs hinted at the soul of the place that had withstood the test of time. I am really sick of seeing those flashing LED signs everywhere these days. The sign looks like it was creatively put together with elements from the old cabins that were salvaged from the fires. The fishing lures and bobbers that dot the sign are also very cute. Someone here has a great deal of creativity. I like the whimsy already. Before entering "the lodge" to get our key, I look over the lake. The water is calm now. There are a few clouds reflected in a darkening twilight sky. Across the lake, I see a bald eagle swirling around a large evergreen. There was always a sign here, always a welcome sign.

The cabins are tidy and modestly appointed. I miss the funkiness of the old linoleum floors, the painted trims, and the Salvation Army furniture of the old cabins, but the new cabins are great. They have been fully restored and rebuilt with a mix of elements of the old cabins and beautiful local hardwoods that were salvaged from the fires. Other updates include energy-efficient appliances, on-demand water heaters to replace those funky gas fixtures and water heaters I remember so well. Our cabin is on the far end of the resort. I believe it is about where Red Oak once stood. That was the first cabin we stayed in with the kids. It was the cabin that tipped inward towards the shore. I remember finding dog toys under the sofa when we left, as everything had a tendency to roll that direction. It is sad to see the treeless hillside behind the cabins, but it is encouraging to see many small trees have taken root there, and a beautiful array of woodland wildflowers dot the hillside. The sunlight that drenches down on the resort now dances with the bright paint colors of the cabins and the wildflowers that surround them. This is a contrast to the shady sunken and faded feeling they had in the past. Late in the day, light spills over the hillside, and there is a pool of colorful reflections in the water—the cabins and their bright new colors.

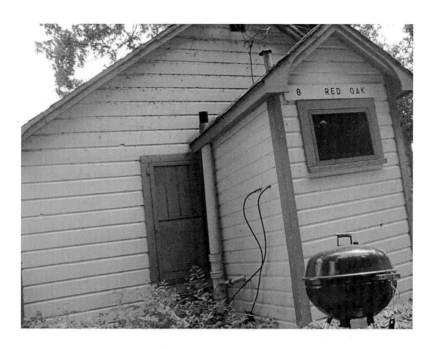

Kassia and Sam met us for dinner tonight. I was very pleased they were able to come up to spend an evening. They were on their way to the UP for another hiking trip. It is nice to have them near us. I am really missing the boys right now. It has been three months since we were last out to see Aleks. I enjoy those little trips to New England, and I am glad I finally have an excuse to visit that part of the country. I was so pleased to see him follow in my footsteps and pursue design and architecture, but I knew he could not turn down the lure of that lucrative MIT scholarship that took him out to the East Coast. His post-graduate work in the design of desalination plants will help solve some of the world's most serious problems. The world could use a few more great minds like his. Our visit this spring coincided with the blooming of the cherry blossoms. We flew into D.C. and headed up to Boston on the train. Aleks has this great apartment with a view of the skyline. The furnishings are slick and modern, and not surprisingly he keeps things very tidy. I can only imagine what he pays in rent. It doesn't seem to matter. He has been able to put away extra money ever since he and Phil came out with those new apps for the iPod. I just downloaded their latest app on Tuesday. This game is a mind-bender, something to keep Mom thinking. He's always had a way of doing that! On top of his projects, it sounds like he has a fun social life, always entertaining or going to concerts. I think he has a special someone out there, but so far, he is keeping the details a secret from his mother. That is okay.

We had a nice visit with Jakoby last month just after his band's CD release party. I am glad we got to see him before the tour. He is now in southern Spain. They have two gigs there before heading over to Ibiza for the One World Concert. There they will open for The Flakes. This is a huge show for them. They are taking a little time after the tour to travel in northern Africa with stops in Morocco, Tunisia, and Algeria. I am so jealous! I've always wanted to go back to Morocco. It is so much easier to travel there now that the Muslim world actually likes us again. Tom and I traveled there in '98 and found it to be such a beautiful and exotic place. What an adventure!

I am glad Jakoby and the band have decided to take time off this fall. Jakoby will be attending law school. His linguistics degree was likely to lead to a life of teaching and academia. This just was not his style. I actually think it was the linguistics background (as well as some challenging life experiences) which added the special poignancy to the lyrics that have caused his band to soar. Law school will be good for him. As a child, he learned the power of debate. He has also had a strong awareness of right from wrong, but most of all, I think it is his compassion and empathy that will serve him in this field. The world could use more lawyers with those qualities. As wild and crazy as his band is, that kid is more tuned in and grounded than anyone I know.

When Kassia and Sam arrived, we were just finishing the final touches on the grilled salmon and fettuccini. Kassia was bringing some strawberries from the farmers market in Madison, so I had also made some of my famous eggless shortcakes.

We set up a table on the deck over the water. I had picked a nice bouquet of wildflowers earlier and used those for a centerpiece. The grills here did not cook the salmon to the perfection of the cedar planks back home, but Tom made this delicious marinade that made up for any shortcomings of the retro-Weber grills that were supplied by the resort. I am still a vegetarian for the most part, but I think I still have a pining for the Pacific Northwest, and I find I can enjoy salmon on occasion especially now that I know there is plenty of fresh native salmon available and that horrible farmed salmon industry imploded in on itself about ten years ago.

We sit down and look out at the water. Tonight, the water is very calm and reflective. In the distance, I hear a couple of frogs and a distant loon. Kassia and Sam seem especially happy and squirmy tonight. I am wondering what is up with them. They tell us about their hiking plans. How they are planning to hike and climb up in the Porcupine Mountains for the next ten days. As we sit down for dessert, Kassia announces they have news they would like to share with us. I watch my daughter... those striking brown eyes... that reassuring smile and dimple. I watch as she tells me they are expecting a baby!

I set my napkin down and without hesitation wrap my arms around her. I lost track of what I said at that point. I know there were tears as I glanced over toward Sam and Tom who were shaking hands and already cracking jokes. I think about the impending diaper duties that are in their future. I collect myself and think for a moment— is my response appropriate? She is only 24 years old. Should I be concerned? In any other situation, I would be, but with Kassia and Sam it is different. Sam is a great guy. They have been dating for 4.5 years now, and he has been such a positive influence on Kassia, such a level-headed guy, a very steady force in her life. This has been a nice balance with Kassia's busy schedule. He keeps her grounded. When Kassia was an undergrad art student at UW-Madison, he was there to see her through those late nights in the studio with all those last-minute projects. He stood beaming next to her at every one of her openings. They are great together, and there is talk of a wedding in the future.

I have no doubt she can handle it with her determination and perseverance. I have seen it in her throughout her life from learning to ride a bicycle in one day. I remember her shouting directions to me over her shoulder as I righted the bicycle when it wobbled. She directed me when to let go, when to hold on, and she soared... and then there was the black belt in martial arts she earned at the young age of 10. She stuck with it and shined as she went through over 300 moves of forms that day. I was so proud. She has always been a planner, an organizer, a juggler. She says she plans to finish up her master's. Her current work intertwines a fine arts degree and art therapy with the UW Medical School. Some of the breakthrough research with neurology and Alzheimer's and art is fascinating. It will certainly help many people. I am so glad she has kept up with her dancing and has a passion she enjoys for herself.

So, I am going to be a grandma! At least for a few years of my life, I thought this was an impossibility. Now I know nothing is truly impossible. Perhaps this is why I am beside myself with excitement right now. I find myself singing as we clean up the dishes and settle in for the night.

CHAPTER 23

"My Doctor Loves Giving Me All This Chemo"

Sent: Tuesday, June 21, 2011

Hi, Mom,

We are just outside of Elgin. The trip was good with only one big downpour around Portage.

We decided to leave Tommy's car at a garage in Madison because it was really acting up. We will retrieve it Saturday. We have a busy evening. I want to get all the laundry done. There were lots of ticks up north found on clothing and such. (Tommy had driven to Fay Lake separately from the rest of the family)

I have to make sure we are stocked up on things because I won't have the car this week when Tommy drives to work. I will let you know how tomorrow goes. I think I will be getting the full four-hour treatment. Starts at 9:20.

We had a great time up there. Fay Lake never seems to disappoint.

Love Stacey

Hi, Mom,

Things are winding down today. They had to. Tommy and I were so stressed. It was a strange 24 hours with the storms, chemo, and the stress of getting everything lined up for that, the broken car, thieves in the night, and then five emergency vehicles showed up next to our house last night—I think they were picking up a drunk or insane walker.

I hung my crystal back up, and I think we need to re-align around here.

We are OK and are seeing opportunities in all of this. Possible job changes, new financial strategies (I found out I can probably get Social Security disability if I want to), or maybe I can get a nice little low-stress job somewhere. Or maybe if Tommy gets a job in the city, we won't need two cars. It will all work out.

I started today with a lavender bath and am staying in my pajamas. Now I am enjoying tea on the front porch. You have a good day!

Love Stacey

Sent: Thursday, June 30, 2011
Subject: hello

Hi, Mom,

The weather has been gorgeous this week, hasn't it? I have not been spending as much time in the garden as you would think, but generally things are looking good. I did a little more planting and moving around in the vegetable garden because there were bare spots.

Things have settled down from last week. We still have not done anything about the car. I actually like being carless. It is nice to keep things simple around here. I am not sure the kids agree. Tommy had some work in the city and took the train in a couple of days this week. That freed up the car for errands. The car shop in Madison will soon get sick of looking at our car, so we must make a decision about what to do about that.

I've been feeling very good since Tuesday. It was a little slow-going through the weekend. Knowing this, I will be more prepared going into my treatment next time. It was a little crazy the night after we got back!

The doctor was very happy that my platelets were stable when I was tested yesterday. Still hanging out in the 70's but not too low. He is weaning me off the prednisone—now only 20 mg every other day. It will be interesting to see if my sleep changes.

I am anxious to hear about your opening. I wish we could have made it up there. I was tired this weekend, and we were still reeling from the car thing and getting back from vacation.

We did attend a feet-in-the-creek day on Saturday that was offered through LivingWell for families. They had some very fun crafts and a nice cookout for us. Then the kids played in a creek. Mom and Dad and Midnight got their feet wet, too! The woman who ran the crafts is also doing a camp for kids on the 13–15 and again in August. I think I will sign the kids up. It is free and she does a really nice job. She does the art classes for their Club Courageous, too.

On Tuesday night we went to a concert in the park. I saw so many friends there—mostly neighbors and former preschool parents. It was a nice night. I like that Elgin has so many free events in the summer.

I've been busy around the house. We painted the front office over the weekend. The color is an auspicious red. I found a computer desk at Goodwill for $14 that I am doing some minor cosmetic repairs on. The room will double as a guest suite when people want to stay. We are putting curtains back on the glass doors, and we will use an arm chair bed in there. It is very pretty! I haven't finished putting art up yet, but I think I will put our Fay Lake watercolors up. That is also where I would like to put up a print of your river painting, and I can also put Grandma's old glass piece on the wall in there.

I am looking forward to Lesley's visit and wanted to get that room mostly finished before she came.

I put up some skateboard decals on Jakoby's wall. I am hoping they stay up—otherwise I will need to paint them. He has fully "christened" the graffiti wall. It looks cool.

Aleks got some little touches for his room at IKEA yesterday. We took a quick outing together while I had the car. His room looks very crisp and nice and clean! He scored an Xbox for $100 yesterday. He was in the market for one and was going to spend $250—all his money—to buy one new. A friend put one on Facebook yesterday, and we snatched it up fast. Now he has enough left over to replace his stolen bike or buy a small flat-screen TV at IKEA. I think he wants to buy a TV assuming Mom and Dad will replace the bike.

For Kassia's room, it is time to get sewing those pillowcases. That and some curtains and some major de-cluttering, and that room should be looking great.

We have some people coming over from We Care today. They are social workers that I guess will come check in and see how we are doing once a month. On Tuesday, I met my "buddy" they teamed me up with. She was very nice. She also has a major chronic illness and has been an unexpected seven-year survivor and is now committed to helping others. I think she will be a good person to talk to. She is coming over on Tuesday mornings each week just to talk and check in. I really feel good about the support we have from all of our family and everyone else. It is such a relief!

I think I will take Midnight for a walk before it gets too warm. We may take our bikes to the farmers market and library later. It could be a scramble because Aleks would have to ride my bike, and I would have to ride Tommy's. We could stop at the waterpark midway for a cooldown if we need it. It could be an adventure, a guaranteed boredom buster. We will see how I feel about it after lunch....

I have a PTA board meeting tonight—grumble grumble... yes, I was elected Enrichment Chairman for next year. I will be organizing the assemblies at Lowrie.

I also should start looking for that "little job." I looked into Social Security benefits and could not qualify for disability due to my spotty work history these last few years. I really did not want to do the SS. It only means that something is coming along, and I will be working and bringing in some income soon!

Love Stacey

Sent: Friday, July 01, 2011
Subject: Tommy

Hi,

Tommy just met with his old company. They want to hire him as Business Development Manager. He is playing cool for now and wants to come back and shoot for either partner or VP of business development maybe in a couple of weeks.

It would be good if he moves into a less stressful environment. The management he is with now seems a little crazy. A pay increase and better benefits would certainly be a plus. I was looking at some paperwork yesterday. Our insurance is nearly $1,300/month. His company contributes less than $400 to that, and we pay the rest.

Stacey

Sent: Saturday, July 02, 2011
Subject: hi

Hi, Mom,

I think I finally slept close to eight hours last night. That felt good. I was very tired yesterday. I went to bed at about 9 p.m. and had a hard time sleeping after 5 a.m., so I got up and wrote, walked the dog, and gardened. A nice way to start a hot, muggy day.

I think we got the first part of the car thing figured out. I signed up for AAA Plus yesterday. They called me with their latest promotion. It comes with 100 miles of towing. We can now chance it on attempting to get the car here next Saturday, and we will have coverage, which we really need anyway. It is much cheaper than a car transport company, which was $300.

Love, Stacey

Sent: Wednesday, July 06, 2011
Subject: hello

Hi, Mom,

It looks like you had a nice 4th of July. I missed that good ol' Boscobel 4th.

We had Robin and Rose over on the 4th and grilled out. It was a beautiful day! Later we lit off all of Tommy's fireworks. That was fun. Once it got dark, we were treated by fireworks displays all around us. It seems that since Elgin did not have a proper display, people went wild with their renegade fireworks.

Tuesday was a lazy day. I was a little tired from the exciting weekend. My new friend came over, and we talked for about an hour. Kassia and I worked on our Costa Rica scrapbooks, finally! That is a fun summer project for us. I took the kids to the library last night once we had the car. We stocked up on some drawing and craft books to keep them busy.

I go in for treatment today. I am taking the bus, so that should be an adventure. It just happens that my appointment time works perfectly with the bus schedule, so we will give that a whirl.

Well, Tommy has his eyes on a used red Saab convertible and a new job. Upwardly mobile or midlife crisis, I don't know! He talked to his old company again yesterday. They are interested. He may be changing within weeks.

I am going to head out and walk Midnight. It is such a nice time of day. I've been getting up early. There are quite a few regular walkers between 6 and 7. My plumber just walked by. I still owe him 125 bucks. I hope he doesn't come by to collect one of these mornings. Hee hee.

I'll let you know how today goes.

Love Stacey

Sent: Saturday, July 09, 2011

Hi, all,

It has been a nice weekend so far. I went to the black belt class last night and then woke up early to help with the labyrinth. We are taking the mulch out and putting in limestone to prevent weed growth. It felt good to pitch in while I was feeling energetic. I shoveled limestone for an hour. It was early (between 8 and 9), so it wasn't too hot. I probably won't do that again, though. My biceps are bulging. :)

Later I had an appointment with Dr. Jaena. I was pretty relaxed after that.

We went to a football sale and got some gear for Aleks. He will start practicing later in the month.

Love, Stacey

Saturday, July 23, 2011
Subject: Tommy

Hi, Mom and Gary,

Tommy is waiting for his official job offer. They want to hire him and actually wanted him to start today. He will probably start in three weeks after reviewing the offer, renegotiating if necessary, and then giving his two weeks' notice. He should get a bump in pay, and we hope the benefits are better.

He worked at this company about six years ago. He seems very excited and relieved.

I feel OK today—just a little headachy. I see Dr. Jaena at 9:20. Maybe she can stick some needles in me and fix the headache.

We had crazy storms last night. Midnight is starting to be afraid of storms. He did not like it. It went on for a couple of hours. The rain is a relief, though.

Stacey

Sent: Monday, July 25, 2011
Subject: Hi

Hi, Mom,

I think Jakoby liked camp. The day did not go as planned, though. I got a call that Kassia had a bad headache. I picked her up at 12:30. She was throwing up, so I took her to the doc after picking Jakoby up. She was diagnosed with an official migraine headache after he checked for other neurological symptoms. She is finally sleeping after quite a bit of suffering.

I am hoping to oil paint tomorrow, but it is probably not likely. I am for sure going to paint next week while they have nature camp. My friend is coming over at 10 a.m. and then Nathan is coming to play in the p.m. I may sneak out to go to the noon Kyuki-do class. It has been more than a week.

I really hope Kassia feels better. It was miserable to see her like that. I am taking her to Dr. Jaena next week. After the first evaluation, kids are free. Love.

Stacey

Sent: Monday, August 08, 2011
Subject: feeling better

Hello there,

I just wanted to let you know I woke up feeling much better today. I am still a little sore, but the overall malaise is gone. I think I will take it very easy today. I started out with a birthday latte and have not moved from my comfortable spot on the sofa.

I really enjoyed the weekend, although I wish I'd felt a little better.

Tommy looked very handsome as he left for his new job. He could not sleep because he was so excited. I am happy for him. I think he feels very good about it. He deserves it! I will talk to you soon!

Love Stacey

Sent: Monday, August 08, 2011
Subject: shitty birthday present

Well, my rain gauge says almost three inches. I think two of it fell in about 15 minutes. The result: our first basement sewer backup ever. Fortunately, it did not extend more than a few feet from the drain. It left Tommy's shower very smelly. We will have to keep the basement picked up now that we know it can happen. It is a big problem in our neighborhood that is being fixed, but it may take a couple of years.

I did some remediation down there and cleared up anything that could get wet. The good thing is, I have two excuses to stay out of the dirty work—it is my birthday and my compromised immune system. :) Poor Tommy.

Stacey

Sent: Tuesday, August 16, 2011
Subject: hello

Hi, Mom,

I have the car just in time to play the role of taxi mom extraordinaire. What a day!

We started by driving to the middle school at 8:20 a.m. to pay fees and get the schedule. I drove across town to get there and then was turned away because I did not have proof of residency. I had already completed registration online, so I never dreamed we would need that. We drove home to get that and then returned with them. What a change middle school will be! They have open house events on Thursday, where we will learn more and get locker assignments.

Once we returned home, my friend Sandy came over at 10 a.m. as she does every Tuesday. After she left at 11, I shot out and did some much-awaited grocery shopping. I got home at 12:40 and was still putting groceries away and feeding the kids lunch when the social workers came over. The minute they left, I had to whisk the kids away and take Aleks to a doctor's appointment.

I had a little chance to sit down, but soon it was time to start dinner. Kassia had to go to a workshop for auditioning at 6 p.m. Aleks decided to hold off on football for a day.

Jakoby and I walked Midnight before I left to pick up Kassia from class just before 8 p.m.

Kassia seems a little apprehensive about the audition, especially after the workshop. I am hoping I can help her boost her confidence. I think she has a pretty good chance of getting in the show (mark your calendar for the weekend of Oct. 7). She auditions tomorrow evening at 6:30 p.m.

I've been feeling reasonably well. I had some reiki yesterday. That felt very good. I did get a rash from the Erbitux. The worst of it has emerged over the last couple of days. I can deal with it. It feels like a sunburn. I think I will go to sleep early today and rest up for another big day tomorrow.

Love Stacey

Sent: Sunday, August 28, 2011
Subject: Re: Hi

The kids should be back in full swing at school this week. Last week was a lot of drilling and getting settled.

Kassia started her practices for the show. It sounds like her part will require lots of dancing. I did get put on the "set" committee. However, it isn't as romantic-sounding as I thought. I will be driving to Cary (20 miles north) on Friday evenings and Saturdays to work in a warehouse with three male team members. The set is being recycled from a previous show but will require some touch-up painting and a few changes. Most of the work will be moving around the large parts and pieces of the set. They were happy to have someone on board who can match paint and do touch-up. I am going to bring a little chair and either play the princess or director role and let the guys move the stuff around. I will jump up with my little paintbrush as needed. I will talk to you soon.

Love Stacey

Sent: Monday, August 29, 2011
Subject: hi

Hi, Mom and Gary,

Aleks came home from practice, and I guess he got MVP for the day. The coach says his tackling is like a Russian bull! My little 80-pounder was tackling this high school kid, I guess.

I thought you would get a kick out of that.

Love Stacey

Sent: Wednesday, August 31, 2011
Subject: today

Hi, Mom,

My treatment went great today. I came well prepared and had everything I needed to be comfortable. I even brought my own fleece blanket because often the air is turned up too high.

They dose me with Benadryl with the new drug, so I usually get sleepy now. I read a little, paged through some magazines and got recipe ideas, listened to the iPod, took a couple of naps, and ate a delicious melon salad and some cheese and crackers.

My doctor seemed very happy with the way things are going. He loves giving me all this chemo! Seriously, he smiled and said, "It seems like we are doing very well." My platelets were 89K today, which is OK. They were 104 last week. He said this confirms that it was probably the oxaliplatin from last year that brought them down and that the other drugs are not affecting it. This leaves us with more options.

I get a little more tired with all the treatments, but it is not bad if I allow myself to rest between stretches of activity. I am actually trying to do light to moderate exercise more often and would like to avoid the hard workouts altogether. The light exercise works well with all the walking to school and dog walks that I am doing now. It was a good feeling to endure the two-hour workout on Sunday, but it took most of my reserves for the next 24 hours, and my muscles were a little sore (I don't think that is good). We did back-to-back forms and kicking combinations for most of the two hours, and in the middle, we had a fitness test. I did 25 push-ups (20, a little break, and then five more), 50 crunchies, and three minutes of jumping jacks.

I decided not to go for the 2nd-degree black belt on November 7. That is a whole story in itself, but I came to the conclusion that I should wait until spring and see if that is a better time. Mainly I don't need the stress (financial or having to perform!).

I have a bowling date with some gals from church tomorrow morning. It should be fun, but I don't know if I will bowl much since I have the pump. We will see how it feels. It will be good to catch up and have some laughs. They are very nice. One of the women is my age, and her husband is facing a similar cancer situation. He's been dealing with it a little longer than me. He just had surgery last week and is doing well. He will start chemo again after recovery.

The rash is getting better after a big breakout this weekend. I don't think that sweat and sunscreen work very well for me right now. I found a Eucerin product that helps. I am going to use this with all of my lovely natural stuff. Hopefully I can keep it to a reasonable level.

That's it for the doctor news. They painted the walls in the treatment room, and I agree with the nurses it is horrible and boring. I admired the fact that they had some nice calming sage green, and slate blue before. Now it is all white and sterile! The fluorescent lights look ten time brighter. I think the designer patient needs to go in and consult, maybe in exchange for a break on some of these copays.... I wonder if they would appreciate my input or be offended. I suppose if sterile is what they wanted, they have it, but even hospitals are getting away from that and are more focused on creating comfortable healing environments.

Love Stacey

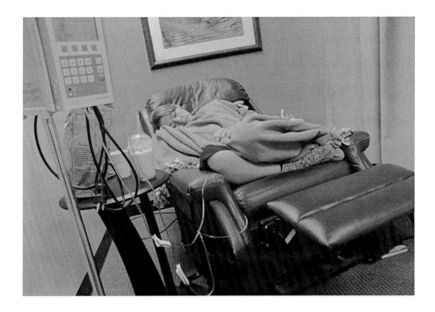

Sent: Monday, September 19, 2011
Subject: Re: Hi

Hi,

I am just finishing a little lunch. It was nice to get an e-mail from you. We had a rainy day yesterday, too. I spent the day at a Dr. Jaena Reboot camp. It was a pleasant refresher. I met some nice people there. Tommy and the kids did some room cleaning and then some errands and football watching.

Saturday, I painted for the sets. There was a warehouse full of busy men working on sets for two shows. I enjoyed myself. I think I am mostly done until everything gets bashed up in the move and needs touch-up again. Kassia got her costume. It is very pretty. The colors are perfect for her—rust and burgundy. Aleks had a football game. He played very well, but they had another loss.

Thursday was Fun Fair. I helped with the face painting. I think I did about 10 snotty little faces! Seriously, it is a joy when they smile at their reflection in the mirror when it is done. Kassia's cupcakes went very quickly. Jakoby clearly had fun. I think he bounced his brains out on the inflatable bounce houses.

I am feeling much better today. I have not been feeling so hot since about last Tuesday. I guess I am due for some fatigue and side effects sooner or later. I am trying my best to slow down and take it easy, alternating rest and activity. On Friday, I am having a maid service come and do an overall cleaning. That will help me tons (would not have been possible without that help from you :)). I cannot imagine what it would be like to have the whole house clean at one time, though I have often fantasized about it. We have slowly been working on our pre-clean this week. I told the kids they have to be able to find your floors in order to clean them. It would be nice to have the beds all washed and done up. I am expecting a new shower curtain and bathroom rug, too. We will be ready for some company.

As for the schedule this afternoon:

4:00—Take Kassia to band sign-up. I think she is going for clarinet with future aspirations of saxophone.

4:45—Take Kassia to theater class.

5:30—Take the boys to football.

6:45—Pick up Kassia from theater class.

8:00—Pick up the boys from football.

I think I will put some chocolate bonbons in my car and some good tunes to make this a pleasant night of taxi service!

Right now, I am going to go get some cheese to make a quick Mexican casserole for dinner. I am also making some stuffed peppers for Tommy and me. It does not look like we will be able to manage any kind of sit-down dinner with this schedule, does it? I at least want to have something made so we don't have to do the take-out thing.

I hope to start my next painting tomorrow. I have an inspiration, and I have a canvas (Hobby Lobby had 40% off last week).

Love Stacey

Sent: Sunday, September 25, 2011
Subject: Bear and Packers

Hi, Mom,

I bet Gary is getting ready for the big game. You should see these boys here dressed in their Bear's jerseys. We are eating our after-church donuts.

Grocery shopping, soup making, and maybe some painting are on my list for this afternoon.

I am feeling better today. My symptoms got worse yesterday, and I almost called the doc or went back, but I decided to wait it out and go on a date with Tommy instead. We went to the Speakeasy and had a good time. The 1.5 glasses of wine and going out must have been what I needed because I am symptom-free today (just a little tired). Go Bears!

Stacey

Sent: Monday, September 26, 2011
Subject: Re: Bear and Packers

Once the Bears were losing, the interest in the game faded. Aleks was in his room playing Madden on his Xbox and Tommy was working on the computer. There was a little hope at the end, though.

I think I broke or sprained some toes last night. I stubbed my foot while getting up to go to the bathroom. Tommy feels bad because he moved a trunk to the end of the bed, and when he did it, I grumbled and said I was going to trip on it someday. Anyway, I went many months without tripping on it, until now. Not being able to walk on it will make the next couple of weeks very interesting. You would not believe our schedule for this theater. Mostly driving back and forth to Huntley.

Stacey

Sent: Monday, September 26, 2011
Subject: hi

We had a very rainy day here. It was relaxing to sit around with my broken toe. I got some computer work done and took a little nap.

I ordered our tickets for the show. I put everyone in one row. We are in the center of the theater about eight or nine rows back, so it should be pretty good.

I got good news from the cleaning service. They are giving me two free cleanings. I signed up for a monthly service. That should be very good. Things have been staying pretty clean around here. Thanks again for helping make that possible.

Love Stacey

Sent: Thursday, September 29, 2011
Subject: hi again

Hi, Mom,

I just got off the phone with you, but I had a couple of other funny stories—probably easier to tell than type, but, oh, well.

After talking to you, I wandered out to my wet little prairie garden. It started raining again. I looked at the rain gauge, and it had overflowed at 5 inches. The next thing I noticed was that our air conditioner was blasting away. I am wearing a jacket in the house, and the air is on. Nice.

The story behind the air conditioner being on started around 5 p.m. yesterday. I was tired from the treatment, mostly because of the Benadryl. It makes me want to sleep, sleep, sleep, even after sleeping almost the whole time I'm there.

I was trying to squeeze in a dinner for the kids before they ran off to their evening activities. Kassia was going to Awana, and Aleks needed a ride to a friend's house across town to work on a project at 6. Jakoby was in and out with his pack of friends.

Suddenly an alarm was going off somewhere in the house. We all walked around trying to find a smoke detector or carbon monoxide alarm that was set off. Just as we would zero in on one, we thought we would hear the alarm coming from somewhere else close by. After going up and down stairs on all three levels, I determined the alarm was coming from somewhere in the attic—either by the furnace or by the fan for our radon unit. I wasn't quite sure what to do, so I started opening windows.

The alarm continued, and I was starting to get a headache (from the noise, I hoped). I spent a little time outside, sitting, we could even hear the alarm out there! I decided I needed to make some calls. I called the radon people to see if there even was an alarm on our system that would be ringing. He did not think we had one installed but suggested it was the furnace or air conditioner. I was getting desperate now. I wasn't quite ready to call the furnace guy and pay a $125 trip fee, so I went to the thermostat and started switching things off and on to see if that would help. Next, I went downstairs to the circuit breaker and started flipping switches. Finally, I sent a desperate IM message to Tommy saying we were leaving the house. I had to drop Aleks off anyway.

We all got in the car. I looked at Aleks and said, "Geez, I can still hear that alarm, can you?"

He said, "Yes," and then suggested it was all just in our heads. We pulled out of the driveway and looked at each other because the sound was still there. Was it coming from the car? NOOOO. I looked down—it was coming from me! My pump had a malfunction, and that obnoxious alarm was attached to me. I was still driving as I began ripping the thing apart assessing which part of the tubing was bent. I nearly ripped it out and threw it out the window. Finally, after stretching out the tube and pushing a button, it stopped and resumed its gentle purr.

Tommy was a little puzzled when he got home and there was no alarm going off, but half of the electricity in the house was not working because I had been messing with the circuit breaker.

The fun never ends here! I was thankful to be able to sit down after going full force between 2:30 and 6:30 last night. I am looking forward to a calm night before our crazy schedule leading into the play. Thursdays are good TV nights.

I wonder how long the air conditioner was on? Love, Stacey

CHAPTER 24
Expect Change

Sent: Thursday, September 28, 2011
Subject: painting

I was thinking about our talk about painting techniques and your "paint-by-number system." I was realizing that I have a distinct methodology to my painting as well, even though it doesn't look like it. I was noticing that it stayed the same even after a long break of no painting. I was wondering if most artists have their own patented methods they follow trained or untrained.

You are a great artist, and I see you getting better and better with each painting. I can't wait to see what you do with Maddie and the butterfly. I just finished a butterfly painting, too—well sort of a butterfly anyway!

Love Stacey

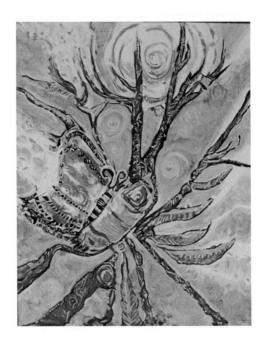

Sent: Wednesday, October 12, 2011
Subject: hello

Hi, Mom,

I had my treatment today, and it went smoothly. I got to sit in the quiet area and read a very interesting magazine from cover to cover, nodding off for only a short time.

I feel much better today. No headache or general aches. I think I sent a message that said no pneumonia.

The doctor did look at my scans and agrees that the lesions on my liver had grown slightly. This correlates with increased CEA as well. I am at 70. He said this still is not high, as he sees numbers in the hundreds and thousands routinely. I was 90 when this whole thing started.

He did not see any additional growth in the lungs or anything new anywhere else. I guess that is about where I thought we were at—perhaps slightly better. I am not alarmed, though I wish it was all good news.

He did not describe it as any of the drugs failing right now. We are continuing to control it so far, just some of the cells are getting sneaky. AND just for the fun of it, he wants to throw ANOTHER drug into the mix (Camptosar). If you are curious and Google it, it would be the FOLFIRI regimen vs. FOLFOX. Both start out with the basic 5FU, but FOLFOX had the oxaliplatin (the nasty drug that killed my platelets and made my hands/feet numb) and the FOLFIRI has the irinotecan (Camptosar). For over a year, I have just been on a reduced version of the 5FU plus Avastin and now Erbitux.

He did not think I would experience drastically different side effects than I am already having. He offered hope of being able to reduce the drug load if I have another nice little remission. :) I think I will think about that.

I think I will go to my yoga class tonight. I don't know if I told you, but I went back to my quiet LivingWell yoga last week. It was very nice. I was happy to see all the familiar faces after about a three-month hiatus. We did a 15-minute guided meditation at the end.

Love Stacey

Sent: Wednesday, October 19, 2011
Subject: Dr. B.

My appointment moved up, which was nice because I then could go there straight from chemo (time/gas saver), and I will be home when the kids get home from school.

I found this doctor very nice, clear, and helpful. He ruled out the possibility of ablation or resection now but did not rule out either further down the road. He agreed with Dr. Y. on the new and continued chemo. If we can shrink and disappear things further, then we will be looking at these as options.

"I have seen this before, and sometimes the drug combinations available now can do amazing things, especially the colon cancer drugs. I have seen miracles." Quote from Dr. B., who is supposed to be black and white and not lead people along with false hopes. He encouraged me to come back each time after I have a scan and he will take a look....

They also offered to show me the scans, which I have never seen before. He showed me the tumors in both lobes of the liver, the right being worse than the left. There is a nice chunk of my liver left lobe that is clear. Ideally what needs to happen is that there needs to be enough shrinkage in one of the lobes (probably the left) so the other lobe could be resected or taken out. If there were small spots left on the section that remains, they could be ablated.

I have my work cut out for me. I need to endure this next round of chemo and keep my other health in check so I am a good candidate for surgery should the day arrive. Thankfully we seem to be doing fine. I will keep doing what I have been doing and then some. I am happy to have the support of so many that allows me to focus on the task at hand! Let's hope for a very special Christmas present.

Stacey

Sent: Wednesday, October 26, 2011

Enjoy your day. Gloomy weather here. I am at treatment. Counts are very good. He is upping the 5FU and adding the new drug. I will likely get a Neulasta shot on Friday to keep my white counts up. I talked to the doctor. Again, he said things only grew a little, but he wants to attack it hard to stabilize. He said we can then cut back. Sounds good to me. Tommy bought me an iPad. He is spoiling me! It is the perfect thing to have here. I have downloaded some of my favorite music, a book (*Walden*), and I will have Aleks help me load a couple of games. I can do Facebook, email, and Internet, too, because they have wireless.

Love Stacey

Sent: Thursday, October 27, 2011

New chemo not so good. I had problems and had to call Jody for a ride home. It was like drinking three hurricanes without the fun part. Dizzy, nausea, slurring... the nurses were helpful and said that can be a side effect if you are not well hydrated. I also think I was anxious. It was kind of like a panic attack. I'm lining up some help for next time. I was fine soon after I got home.

Today I am nurturing myself. Lots of water and a good breakfast so far. Can't say we will do a dog walk, but the sun is poking through, and it is tempting.

Love Stacey

Sent: Tuesday, November 01, 2011
Subject: Hospital

I was admitted to the hospital tonight. This time for GI issues. Some tests tomorrow and maybe a colonoscopy. Will be glad to get it all figured out. I guess it's a dramatic way to get the docs all working together.

I'm feeling better than earlier this week and would rather be raking leaves tomorrow. I will stay in touch. Love ya.

Stacey

Sent: Wednesday, November 02, 2011
Subject: Hello

Hi, all,

Just a quick update... I know some of you got bits and pieces.

The scope revealed inflammation, a lot of which was at my previous surgery site. The doc here is calling it colitis, the likely result of one of my chemo drugs. They are keeping me longer because they wanted to rule out infection, and I have diarrhea—possibly from an antibiotic given to me earlier in the week or a side effect of the CPT 11. I could not have ridden this one out safely at home. I am being given fluids and potassium tonight as well as a different antibiotic. Tom has been working from home. His new company seems very good about that. Friends and neighbors have offered to help with rides, child care, and meals if needed. Thanks for all of your thoughts and wishes.

I don't think they are too worried about me here. If I see a nurse once every 2-3 hours, I am lucky.

I think they are afraid of me now because I really let loose when they said my liquid diet will be maintained until sometime tomorrow. I am drinking chamomile tea and have that fantastic lavender from Community Pharmacy. I plan to sleep tonight and dream of that veggie burger....

Love to all of you, Stacey

Sent: Saturday, November 05, 2011
Subject: Growing up

Hi, Mom,

Well, I think I am starting to have a teenager on my hands. Last night Aleks asked to go to a "party." I asked whose party, and he did not give me a name—only said it was a girl's who went to his school. "What kind of party?" I asked. "I don't know, but I think they are having a bonfire. Paulie and Max are going," he said. I said if he really wanted to go, I could call Paulie's mom to get more info. Later I found Paulie wasn't going. He did not push it too hard, but I got a taste for what it will be like. Much too early for that.

Today he was telling me about a new rotation at school. He is taking a cooking class. That will come in handy. :)

Love, Stacey

A Vacation to Florida in January 2012

Sent: Sunday, January 01, 2012
Subject: Air-bound

Happy New Year! We are in flight. So far things are going well. We got to the gate as it was boarding. Turbulence ahead, I guess. I am anxious for the coffee cart. We got up at 4 a.m.

Hope you had a fun night. I woke at midnight and went downstairs. Aleks wanted to get up. He stayed in his room and texted. I watched some fireworks—there were many in the neighborhood.

Some even landed on our roof. Tommy slept through it.

We should be on the beach by 3 p.m. We will let you know when we arrive safely.

Love Stacey

Sent: Sunday, January 01, 2012
Subject: Neptune

Hello,

We got here, and the weather was beautiful. It will get much cooler on Tuesday.

Ate at Nervous Nellie's. They had outdoor seating on the water and a live reggae band. It was a good place to get in the vacation mood while waiting for the room. The Neptune is great. It seems pretty full. The kids swam—nice beach, and a beautiful first sunset for 2012. Tom and the kids went to get groceries. I am ready to snuggle in and read. Hope all is well.

Love Stacey

Sent: Monday, January 02, 2012
Subject: Re: Neptune

Nice morning. Jakoby found hermit crabs. I went for a morning walk and got some breakfast while everyone was sleeping. Glad we got an early start because it was sunny and 72, but it is changing fast. We should still have plenty of sun and warmer temps by end of week.

Stacey

Sent: Tuesday, January 03, 2012
Subject: Baby it's cold outside

I just spent an hour by the pool with the kids. I had four layers on, jeans, and stocking cap. They were swimming—the wind chill is 45. They did not seem to mind until they got out.

Maybe we will go see manatees later. I guess they are all coming in to the warm waters, and people are flocking to see them. I think I am done with the pool and beach for today!

Stacey

Sent: Wednesday, January 25, 2012
Subject: Re: Hi

Hi,

The doctor was fine today. It was quick and uneventful. No new suggestions for the belly. I don't think they are too worried. I see my GI doc on Monday anyway for a general follow-up.

I had lunch with Jennifer after my treatment. We went to The Neighborhood Deli. I had my usual egg salad and some spicy Thai spinach/peanut soup as well as a brownie.

Tommy thought the class intro was good last night. We will be putting Aleks through 28 hours of Sex Ed training. They make it fun and schedule it as a once-a-month supervised co-ed sleepover event with tons of snacks.

We got an early April's fool joke from Blue Cross in the mail—letters saying our policy was terminated in November. Along with it came a statement for one of my medical encounters that said, "You may owe the provider $11,543." I was not too worried about it, knowing that I had claims after that date that were accepted. I guess Tommy found out this letter was accidentally sent to all employees at his company. Interesting.

I may try to go to yoga tonight. I haven't been in a while, because of the holidays and vacation.

Tomorrow I have a free reiki session at LivingWell. In addition, the We Care people are sending me my own personal masseuse, a Hispanic male with strong hands. I had to get clearance from Tommy. He thought it sounded great and was happy the service was available. What a sweetie, not the jealous type. I might get the neighbors talking, though. Ah, the cancer perks....

A little lingering tiredness from the Benadryl today. That stuff really hits me! A little nap would be nice right now. I have some party preparations to work on. It should be a full weekend.

Love Stacey

Sent: Friday, January 27, 2012
Subject: Re: Hello

I got my massage with Arturo lined up for Monday. I will let you know how it goes.

I am very excited about the party weekend. Jakoby is having three boys over for a sleepover tomorrow. We will start by taking them to Epic Air Trampoline Park. Hopefully they will burn off some energy there! After that, we will have pizza and cake. I might get an oblong pan and try to make a turtle. It shouldn't be too hard. The boys will watch a movie, play video games, and hopefully sleep a little. I still have to get him a birthday present.

On Sunday we are cooking our Christmas turkey. Jakoby is excited about having a feast for his birthday.

I just talked to Tommy, and he had some shocking news about one of his closest coworkers who practically runs the company. They just found a mass in his colon. He is 45. Tommy offered his support but also is respecting his privacy. I hope I can be of help if he needs it.

Tommy is having an endoscopy on the 14th because he is having reflux problems that are getting worse. He was fully scoped and clean three years ago, so I am not too worried. He had irritation in his esophagus back then which they speculate could be the cause related to stress.

I am going to clean a little for tomorrow. Man, my energy just hasn't stopped in the last couple of days. I am happy for that. Midnight is, too. He got another long walk today. I will remember to take it easy... we don't want a repeat of the last birthday.

Love Stacey

Sent: Monday, January 30, 2012
Subject: Hi

Hi, Mom,

The doctor's appointment today went really well, and so did the massage. Arturo was a very nice man. He will be coming every week, and he left his massage table here so Tommy and I can give each other massages. He said he does not use it right now. Tommy was very excited. The gastroenterologist did not think my stomach looked bad now. He had some good advice for diet and supplements. He and my oncologist have been talking about me behind the scenes. I got a better sense of what they are thinking and about my treatment plan. It sounds like it will be on and off, and the oncologist will be monitoring side effects closely. I like the way they are communicating and the fact that I am not just a number. These are two very busy doctors.

Jakoby had a birthday hangover and stayed home today. Just a little tummy upset.

Love Stacey

Sent: Wednesday, February 01, 2012
Subject: Hi

Hi, Mom,

Things went so smoothly today, at least up until 3. I got in to the doctor early and got done before the kids got home.

Kassia had an after-school program, and I had Jakoby set up to go to Trevor's. I figured I had an extra hour to rest before they got home. When I laid down, I realized the nurses forgot to put the large bandage over the site where the needle goes in for my pump. This could be a problem because it could pop out while I sleep, or it could get wet with bathing. I had to line up a return trip to my doctor's office to have that done. Fortunately, another friend was able to swing by and take me out there. All the kids were getting out at the various schools on the way, and I did not feel comfortable driving.

My doctor was super impressed by those numbers today. When I saw the spike two weeks ago, I was a little scared, but something told me there was a reaction going on (especially with the fever) and that it might not be all bad. He brought the chart to me and said I should frame it and gave me the biggest hug. If the trend continues, I will be at zero in two weeks. I like his plan about doing a PET scan after a couple more treatments.

Thanks for offering to help with the big treatments. I would say that so far, I am adapting, though it is a little harder than it was before. Your help, love, and good company are always appreciated. I really enjoyed our last visit. I would just plan it for a time which is easy on you. I don't want to say it, but if I ever had to go to the hospital, that is when I would need the most help.

I have a few lazy days planned. I may paint tomorrow or the next day. :) Have you done any painting? Love, Stacey

Sent: Wednesday, February 15, 2012
Subject: Hi

Treatment went pretty well today. My counts were all OK. I met another really nice lady there named Maria. A couple of my other Wednesday friends were there. I talked briefly to the Mexican guy's sister (they were there when you were). I don't think he is doing very well.

I talked to my doctor briefly, and he said we should talk next week about the plan. I am sure he will want to see the latest CEA, which I think they took today. He said he would really like to give me a break. I hope we find a good reason to have one!

Tommy's boss had surgery and is recovering and working on figuring out next steps. It sounds like he is stage 3, so he will probably do chemo for a while. He has a big family. Tommy says 6 or 10 kids, ages 6–20. I think I will write him a note so he can e-mail me with questions. It sounds like he is taking it pretty well.

I've got my tummy back, and I mean MY tummy. The pudgy little tummy where I can grab a couple inches of flab—not the pregnant belly. That digestive stuff that was done last week was intense but really helped. I have continued to lose some weight but hopefully can gain some back if the digestive tract is healing.

I am looking forward to a few lazy days. I don't have any commitments but hope to get out and do some walking as the weather warms. It felt rather spring-like today. How's your week going? Love, Stacey

Sent: Wednesday, February 29, 2012
Subject: Treatment update

Hi, all,

I just finished one of my big treatments. Blood counts were very good—a relief because I have two sick kids. Kassia stayed home with another stomach flu, and Aleks has a bad cough. I most likely will skip the white count shot on Friday. I should feel better sooner as a result.

They tried to do the treatment without Benadryl because it was making me dopey. (I actually like the dopey during treatment!). I felt nauseous and thought my heart was racing, so they ended up giving it to me after all. Things went much better after that.

Jody picked me up, and it was so windy outside I could barely stand. My scarf blew off my head, and I had to go running after it through the parking lot. Very comical. It would have been in the middle of Randall Road in no time.

I talked to my doctor, and this is the latest plan… I will have a CT scan next Thursday. He wants to get Dr. B. involved. He feels he needs an apples-to-apples comparison to study the scans, so no PET scan just yet. He said he wants to look into ablation. They have a new drug or chemical that is working much better. If Dr. B. feels a PET scan would be advantageous, they will do that, too.

I am happy with the plan. I keep thinking about the road sign yesterday—"expect change." I think I will interject "expect good change" and go with that. Maybe the driving will be rougher around here, but a little less chemo would be a good change.

Hope all is well in Wisconsin. I may be seeing some of you next weekend.

Love Stacey

From: Thomas Lesiewicz
Sent: Thursday, March 01, 2012
To: Stacey Reynolds
Subject: Re: Drug

Have I ever told you how much I love you?

Sent: Friday, March 02, 2012
Subject: Re: Drug

Well, I spent three hours obsessing over the wrong drug. So, it is not the PV-10 for now. I had a brief moment to talk to my doctor today, and he said it was the radiofrequency ablation he was looking into. The new more effective drug or compound is called imetrium (spelling is not correct because I can't Google it). He was cautious in telling me they have to be able to get to the lesions to do the procedure and that is why they are running the scans. This scares me a little because I know I may have one in a tricky spot. I did read they can "open you up" and do the procedure to get around that.

The laparoscopic procedure is usually well tolerated with a little pain and sometimes flu-like symptoms for 7–10 days. It can be repeated as necessary.

The PV-10 does sound interesting and may be something very promising around the corner. I will ask the liver doctor about it because I am sure he is very familiar with it and what stage of approval it is in.

Tommy is going to be an advocate, and we will push so all options are considered. I know this liver doctor is one of the best and can probably do some riskier and more complicated things. He was part of a team of doctors for Mother Teresa. Can you beat that?

CT scan next Thursday. Initial results the following week. Talk to you soon,

Love, Stacey

Wednesday, March 07, 2012
Subject: Aleks FB post

Aleks' algebra teacher was recently diagnosed with cancer and had surgery. I found out from his Facebook post that she just passed away. He talked to me about it this a.m. and seems a little sad but is OK. He showed me his text stream, and I guess all the kids are posting their RIPs. I am sure they will have a counselor come in or something.

Stacey

CHAPTER 25

Each Day Is a Blessing

Sent: Wednesday, March 14, 2012
Subject: Today

Hi, all,

Had my big treatment. Maybe my last one for a while. Not all good news, though...There was some small progression in both lungs and liver. Doctor still describes it as being controlled, but the cancer cells are getting smart. There is nothing new showing up, so that is very good!

He is going to do more research but thinks he will put me on an oral pill chemotherapy treatment called Xeloda. We need to change things up a little to trick the cancer. The regimen is that I will take a pill for two weeks and then have one week off. I will probably still go in for Erbitux weekly, and he may reintroduce Avastin on and off. Not a candidate for ablation right now in his opinion.

Taking the news with mixed reaction. It's just part of the journey with its ups and downs, and it has been a pretty smooth ride for me so far. Not as good as I hoped, but not as bad as it could be. I am doing fine and can't tell you how grateful I am for everybody and everything. Each day is a blessing.

And you better believe I will be enjoying the next week with the forecast! Hope you will, too. Call me any time.

Love Stacey

From: Carole Young
Sent: Wednesday, March 14, 2012
Subject: RE: Today

Hi, Stacey,

You are a beautiful person, and I hope you know I am on this journey with you. Love you so much.

Laurie filled me in about your weekend. I'm glad you girls and the cousins could get together for some sister time.

Yes, I am enjoying the early spring, too.

Love, Mom

Sent: Thursday, March 15, 2012
Subject: Re: Hi

I am just resting upstairs after a pretty busy day and a big evening coming up.

The social worker from We Care is here with the kids. The kids are playing Twister.

I had a dog walk, a meeting, lunch with Jennifer, and just a little raking so far. This evening Kassia has her first art opening at a bank. I just found out about it an hour ago. That will take the place of the PTA meeting I was going to. Not able to do both—lucky I am out at all. I will send pics of the art opening. Tommy will be taking Aleks to a career night at the middle school. Never too early to start thinking about jobs, right?

Would love to talk soon. I'd call, but I might catch you in that nice bath. I might try to close my eyes for a few minutes here and then put something cheery on for the opening.

Tomorrow is a good day for calls. I run in to the doctor to get this pump off at 8:50, and then I am free and probably free of this pump apparatus for a long time. Yippee!

Love Stacey

From: Lesley Reynolds
Sent: Thursday, March 15, 2012
Subject: phone call

Hi, Mom.

I'm sorry I didn't have much to say today when you asked me what I thought about Stacey's email. I guess I felt like I didn't know what to say. I am thankful that things aren't worse and that her attitude is so incredible, but also worried.

I guess I just wanted to tell you I don't want you to feel like you can't talk to me about things if you ever feel like you need to. I may not have much to say, but I'm a pretty good listener.

That's all for now. Time for a movie and some beer and chips and guacamole.

It got up to 81 here today! I wish I had a space to garden. I think I'd take my chances on a little crop of spinach or salad mix. Talk to you soon.

Lesley

From: Carole Young
Sent: Thursday, March 15, 2012
To: Lesley Reynolds
Subject: RE: phone call

I didn't think you should talk about it more than you did. It's a hard thing for all of us. I appreciate that Stacey always tells me exactly how it is. At least I think she does. I worry about her, but I always feel better after I talk to her.

Love, Mom

Sent: Wednesday, March 21, 2012
Subject: pv-10 and doctor

Hi, all. Happy spring!

This is a follow-up to my e-mail about obsessing over the PV-10. I wrote my doctor a note and asked him to please look into the progress on that drug. Today when I went in, he said he wanted to talk to me about it—he had something to tell me. He actually got my hopes up a little. He told me he was very familiar with that drug. He is aware of the stages of clinical trials going on and all of that. It just is not quite there yet, and it may be awhile. He did reassure me that if anything does happen, he will let me know about it. We have a little more work to do with the chemo (and wheatgrass juice) anyway.

I start the Xeloda tomorrow. I am going to put that little bottle of pills in a place where they will soak up some good energy. Hopeful and apprehensive.

Tommy has his endoscopy tomorrow. He is looking forward to a big burrito for lunch when that is done.

I am doing a Dr. Jaena retreat this weekend. It is just Saturday and Sunday with no overnight. I think that it will be timely.

I hope you are all getting out and enjoying the weather. I have found it very energizing. I can't decide whether I am ahead or behind on the yardwork. I got an early start, but things are moving along so fast it is getting ahead of me. I have some asparagus to eat tomorrow. :) My first edible, unless you count my parsley which wintered over—uncovered, in a container.

Lots of love, Stacey

Hi, all,

Everything was fine with the endoscopy. The doc said everything looks good. Tommy Is in recovery and is enjoying the meds. We will probably go out for lunch after he sleeps them off a bit. He is really funny right now.

I am doing fine with the Xeloda. I am trying to do it without anti-nausea meds. I am actually a little extra hungry right now.

Love Stacey

Sent: Thursday, March 29, 2012
Subject: Weekend

Hi, Mom,

Still no decision about the weekend. We are both feeling a little tired and overwhelmed this evening. House is a mess, lots of yardwork to do, mowing, fertilize, raking, bills to pay, mountain of laundry... Eeks!

My energy is coming in small spurts. Maybe we will reenergize overnight and have a different perspective tomorrow. Tommy is going to a Buddhist meditation group through church tonight. He always teases his mom about becoming Buddhist.

Love Stacey

Sent: Friday, March 30, 2012
Subject: Aargh

Hi, Mom,

I did not have the greatest night. I was up running to the bathroom. Things settled down about 1 a.m. Later we had thunderstorms, and Midnight was scared and was climbing and panting all over me. I am at the doctor getting fluids. I don't feel too bad, and everything checks out good. I even weighed more than Wednesday. I just did not want to end up in the hospital if it happened again.

Anyway, things are not boding well for the weekend unless I can get a good night of sleep and nip this little problem in the bud. I will let you know what is going on. I may take a little nap while I am here. The kids will want to paint this afternoon. Tommy is working from home on Fridays now, so that is nice.

Love, Stacey

Date: Fri, 30 Mar 2012
Subject: Re: Aargh

Hi, Mom,

I don't think we will be able to come. I am feeling OK, but, feel like I need to rest and get caught up. Tom is traveling two days next week, so I want to make sure everything is in line. I am having some issues come up again this evening after a symptom-free day. I just took a nice big dose of Imodium, so let's hope that does the job.

The doctor wanted to prescribe Prostatin, but I had my iPad and Googled the side effects, and the first two were diarrhea and gas. What the heck? I said I will try to make a go of it with the Imodium and declined the drug. He seems like he wants to keep me on the high dose of Xeloda. I will talk to you soon.

Love, Stacey

Sent: Sunday, April 01, 2012
Subject: Re: Aargh

Hi, Mom,

Well, so much for catching up. I spent much of yesterday in bed. At least I finally finished *Harry Potter 4*.

I am still having some issues. It was pretty bad again last night. It is good we did not come because I was up a couple of times in the night, and the evening was bad. I will probably check in with the doctor tomorrow, but I think I can avoid it today as long as I drink lots of water. Tommy is going to do some grocery shopping and fold some laundry. If the sun does come out, I will try to get out in the yard a little. That might help my spirits at least.

Back to school for the kids tomorrow. I think they had a fun spring break. Have a good day.

Love Stacey

Sent: Tuesday, April 03, 2012
Subject: cancer fundraisers

Hello, all,

Aleks is collecting money for Kimball Kares. This is the fourth year for the event, which raises cancer awareness among students and collects donations which go to local cancer centers and to a staff member affected by cancer. It is a special year for the event because one of the main organizers, Mrs. Jones (Aleks' algebra teacher), recently passed away from cancer. The school is hoping to raise $2,000.

I am sure that Aleks would be happy with even the smallest donation towards the cause and would feel like he was making a difference. Let us know if you can help—even $5 is OK. I think it is due Friday.

On another related note, I plan to do the American Cancer Society Elgin Walk and Roll on May 4th. I feel good about my ability to do the walk as long as I can resolve this most recent little problem of mine. I want to get my "third" survivor shirt from the walk this year, and of course I want to do what I can to raise money to help others. I will send the link in an upcoming e-mail. Thank you if you've already donated.

Love Stacey

Sent: Tuesday, April 03, 2012
Subject: Re: cancer fundraisers

I was fine today until the monster hit at about 1:30. I enjoyed the beautiful day and walked Midnight, did some gardening, and talked to some neighbors. I was out of commission for the rest of the afternoon and evening. It is a good thing I go in tomorrow because it is getting worse each day. I don't think I am too dehydrated, but I am definitely losing weight. I will get some medicine, fluids, and then I will have my week break. I called today, and they said just keep drinking lots of water, and they will assess me when I come in.

Did you have nice weather there? I planted my broccoli seedlings and transplanted my tomato seedlings to larger containers. Other than that, I started to clean up the flower/strawberry garden next to the driveway. I have strawberry blossoms and blossoms on my apple tree. The picture of us by the tree last year was taken in early May when it was blossoming.

I look forward to seeing Lesley. It looks like it will be a pretty good weekend. I sure hope I get this problem cleared up by then. Talk to you soon.

Love Stacey

Sent: Wednesday, April 04, 2012
Subject: Pain in the a__

Hi, Mom,

Everything went well today. I got the Sandostatin. They did not tell me it was going to be a big shot in the behind. It is long-lasting and is only needed once a month. I expect to be a little sore from the injection and am looking forward to it working after about two days. So far, symptoms today do not seem quite as bad as yesterday. I feel like resting tonight. I bought some frozen pizza for dinner. I will keep you posted. Everything seems good for now.

Love Stacey

Sent: Thursday, April 05, 2012
Subject: Thanks for donations

Hello,

Thanks for the donations for Kimball Kares. Aleks told me when he got in the car that the office staff was very happy when he brought in a check for $100. I think the event is very important to the school this year because everyone has been touched by cancer with the loss of one of their favorite teachers. Aleks seemed very happy to contribute. :) Love, Stacey

Sent: Friday, April 06, 2012
Subject: Fay Lake reservations

Hi,

We are booked for June 15, 16, and 17 at Fay Lake. We rented half of the townhouse this time for something new. It should be fun. The kids have been asking about it.

Tommy is taking Fridays off for long weekends this summer instead of longer duration chunks. We will probably do shorter trips close to home (or SW Wisconsin!) for the remainder of the summer.

I took the kids to breakfast while the maids cleaned this morning. A life of luxury I lead...

I don't feel so hot today—stomach cramps and tired. I am taking it real easy so I can enjoy the weekend. That new medicine is supposed to kick in soon.

Love Stacey

Sent: Tuesday, April 10, 2012
Subject: No news good news?

I didn't hear anything from the doctor today, so that is probably good. I have my appointment at 9:20 tomorrow. Doubt I will be doing any treatment. Symptoms have improved but are not gone. I ate more today and got out and went to Trader Joe's. Pretty low on energy, though. That is OK if I get a couple of things done in the morning and then have a lazy afternoon.

We got picked for a rain garden! I really did not think we had a chance. They have to check for utilities underground because they dig more than 12 inches deep.

Stacey

Sent: Wednesday, April 11, 2012
Subject: Doctor

My blood counts were great! Love that green juice.

Still waiting on culture results. The nurse did say it can be treated outpatient if there is an infection. I will get Erbitux today. I get another week break from Xeloda, and the dosage will be reduced. I will also be taking potassium and magnesium supplements.

I feel a little better today, just very tired... they said because of the mineral loss.

Huge weight loss this week—disappointing but no surprise. I need to find that box of size fours or go on a little shopping trip. ;)

They are running slow today. I will be here until the kids get home at this rate. I better get my nap in when the Benadryl hits.

Love Stacey

Sent: Thursday, April 12, 2012
Subject: Today

Hi, Mom,

I spent the morning chilling out at Dr. Jaena's office. That was nice. I then went to the thrift store to buy some size 4 jeans. Tommy said I don't have to shop at the thrift store, but for jeans that I plan to grow out of soon, it makes sense. Once home, I took Midnight on a much-needed walk. It was a beautiful day. I am so happy the light frost last night did not damage the blossoms. I covered my strawberries but probably did not need to.

Later I got some yardwork done. I raked some piles of leaves. I hope I can get them bagged before the rain comes tomorrow. It sounds like we will get quite a bit of rain over the weekend. That will be good for weeding next week, and oh, boy, do I have weeds.

I probably will take it easier tomorrow, but it is good knowing my old energy is coming back. I just have to keep up with these fluids and mineral supplements. I wish the other part would go away, too.

Still did not hear the lab results so I am once again assuming that is good. I will talk to you soon.

Love Stacey

Sent: Friday, April 13, 2012
Subject: Re: Weight

Hi, Mom,

I just went to get fluids because I called in and the nurse said to just do it after I ran through my symptoms. I did not want to have to do it at the ER over the weekend, and I want to feel good. It is cheaper to pay the co-pay at my doc's office—$40 ($150 for ER). I also have more interesting things to do than sit in the ER for six hours, and there's always the risk that they will admit me.

The weather was turning when I got home. It was cloudy and breezy, but I did go out and get the leaves raked into bags.

I got hit with my affliction at about 2 p.m. So that issue is not over. There were slight signs of improvement this morning.

Tomorrow is a busy day. We have two seats for a breakfast and wildflower walk at 9 a.m. from the church auction.

Kassia has science fair at the library in the morning, and Aleks has it in the afternoon. We are still waiting to see how things are looking in the morning, but I think Jakoby will be my date for the breakfast. I am looking forward to it because they are very good hosts, and I know the food will be great. If we go on the walk, I am sure Jakoby will enjoy some info about the frogs and turtles in the forest preserve there.

I am hoping for a weekend of healing and renewal. Tomorrow will be busy, but I think we will have a lazy Sunday. Maybe I will give you a call.

Love Stacey

Sent: Monday, April 16, 2012

Hi, Mom,

The doctor turned out fine today. I have no icky infections. I got another prescription to help with my symptoms. I will go back on the Xeloda at half the dose I was on beginning Thursday. Everything else is looking good. I am feeling OK.

I think we might try to come on that weekend of the 28th pending everything. Just plan on the possibility. :)

Sent: Tuesday, April 17, 2012
Subject: Aargh

Hi,

I got a call this a.m. that both my potassium and magnesium were too low. I have to go to Sherman to get an infusion. It will take five hours, so I will spend the afternoon here. I was out early this morning buying potting soil for gardening this afternoon. Boo hoo. Klein's opens tomorrow, and I want to be ready to plant those flowers. Oh, well. Home around five. I will call the school so Kassia knows and will call and check on them at 2:45.

Love Stacey

Sent: Tuesday, April 17, 2012
Subject: Re: Aargh

I am home and fine. Tummy is much better today, so I should not have to do that again. The new prescription did the trick. I will plant tomorrow as long as I am not at the doctor too long. Not too early to pot pansies and Johnny Jump-Ups. They can survive light snow or frost. That is all I will do for now. Had a relaxing afternoon.

Love Stacey

Sent: Monday, April 23, 2012
Subject: Hi

Hi, Mom,

Waited forever to see my doc. I guess I am glad I went, though. I read about this horrible toxic mega colon thing on the Internet and thought I should rule that out. I will be in touch with and see the doctor on Wednesday. He may order a CT to rule out fluid build-up. He did not think I sounded very fluidy, though. Up to 134 lbs. again! I am all over the place. Potassium was still a little low.

I hate to say it, but I think the diarrhea is back. I am pretty certain we will see improvement in my girth over the next couple of days.

Ok, I need a day or two of not talking about BM. Something is telling me to go plant some flowers this week, finish the book I am reading, and go to Whole Foods and explore a new recipe.

Love Stacey

Sent: Thursday, April 26, 2012
Subject: Hello

Hi, Mom,

I just wanted to check in with you. I had my scan today, but no results yet. I am fine either way but am hoping it is digestion. I should know tomorrow sometime.

I had the greatest day! I got up early and started clearing clutter in the dining room. The bookshelf had papers hanging off of it. It wasn't long before I had piles all over the place. It became quite a project. Next, I was rearranging plants and artwork and setting everything just right. It looks a lot better.

I made myself a yummy little tofu scramble for breakfast.

I called to move my scan forward. I thought it would be nice to have results before the weekend, so that was at 11:45.

I went to Kathy's for our weekly coffee date. The other two friends were busy. So, it was just the two of us. It was nice to catch up with her.

After the scan, I decided to stop at the ReStore on the way home. I haven't been there in a couple of years, so I just wanted to scope things out. I looked at some light fixtures, carpet, and ceramic tile. On the way out, I ran into this dining room table that was very large and very solid-looking. Now this is something we really need! A table we can actually put a meal on and get at least five chairs around. Better yet, one that could accommodate guests. It was new and a very good deal. I checked with Tommy and snagged the deal. It is so strange this fell into place after spending the early morning organizing the dining room—it was meant to be. We will have to work on chairs, but it is a great table—very architectural and substantial and solid wood. We have to rent a U-Haul to bring it home on Saturday because they don't do deliveries.

After the kids came home, I went to my Dr. Jaena appointment. I felt great afterwards. All of these treatments this week have been helping out immensely.

I made some good homemade pizza for dinner.

It was a busy evening. Tommy went to his Buddhist meditation. I had the privilege of driving Aleks to his dance. What a feeling to see my once little guy leap from the car, cell phone in hand. So big and independent. I picked him up at 8 p.m. He said the music was very loud. It looked like a well-attended dance. The parking lot at pickup time was a zoo.

As you can probably tell, my energy is gradually picking up. My back is still achy from the extra weight. The warm pad helps with that when I can sit.

I think I will take it easy tomorrow. Maybe the declutter streak will continue.

Thank you for the donation for the walk. That made my day too! I took that as a message that I will get myself in shape over the next week so I can do it. I will show up for it one way or another. I really appreciate the support from you and everyone else. It means so much to me. Such an important cause.

Tommy and I are going out for a much-needed date night on Saturday.

Love Stacey

Sent: Friday, April 27, 2012
Subject: Results of scan

I have not talked to my doctor yet, but I did pick up the results today. The report was more detailed than expected.

Here's what I know. I will avoid too much speculation until I talk to Dr. Y.

Good news: Once again, nothing is showing up anywhere else. So, there is nothing new to worry about. The report also said that the majority of mets appeared stable.

Bad news: I have a moderate to large amount of fluid build-up. Cause? My doctor has already discussed using a catheter to drain this. He does not want to do water pills because my potassium would be further depleted. I don't know what this involves yet (inpatient/outpatient), but I am sure it will happen next week.

Four spots on my liver are larger, and my liver is slightly enlarged.

I found out Wednesday that my CEA was in an upward pattern.

Good, good news: I have been very energetic the last two days in spite of some aches and discomfort from the swelling. While I would rather the report was better, I am encouraged by my ability to regain my energy and strength back from a couple of weeks ago, and my appetite is great.

The rest of my bloodwork has been relatively good. In fact, my liver enzymes had gone down nicely.

I am putting this in perspective and focusing on two things: 1. Getting rid of this fluid so I can be more comfortable. 2. I am obsessed about doing something about those four spots and will grill the doc because this time it says other areas are stable. I am willing to risk it and go off chemo for a while to treat these areas if it is still possible.

So that is what I know. Now, I am not sure about the walk. I am physically taking it easy because I know a lot of walking will make this head down to my feet. I have already talked to Kassia and her friend Nicole about walking in my place. I will go to see them off and see them come in.

Looking forward to a lazy weekend. I just stocked up at Trader Joe's. We get our new table tomorrow afternoon (my ReStore find). Yeah!

Tommy and I are going on a date night tomorrow night, yeah! I decided it couldn't be a fancy dinner place because I might be stuck wearing my yoga pants. Prairie Rock re-opened. Maybe we can try that. Perhaps a movie, too.

On Sunday, we will grill out or cook a big chicken dinner and see how much food we can get on that table!

You all have a good weekend. Call me if you wish. I should be around most of the weekend.

Love Stacey

Sent: Monday, April 30, 2012
Subject: Hi

Hi, Mom,

Had a pretty good weekend. It was a little lazy because I was trying to stay off my feet.

The date night was wonderful. We needed that.

We have been enjoying the table. What a difference it makes. There has been some major Monopoly action going on around here.

I called the doc first thing to see what we could do about getting this paracentesis scheduled. I just spoke to him, and he is going to call to have it ASAP—maybe tomorrow, as I said I was flexible about which hospital it is done at.

I read about the process, and it sounds like it is only an hour. (Make that four with registration, prep, and recovery.) Not a big deal. The doctor said they will leave a catheter in because they will likely need to repeat. Yuck. I will just be happy to be able to resume my gardening and such, not to mention wear my clothes again.

I am seriously considering sending the kids to Sugar Creek again. I have to talk to Tommy, but I think the experience would be good for them. One week that looks good is July 8. That is before football gets all hot and heavy, and they have programs for all three that week. Are you around that week? We can hang out or whatever, depending on what my treatment status is then. Fun. :) I hope you are having a good visit and are getting your garage sale together. Talk to you soon.

Love Stacey

Sent: Tuesday, May 01, 2012
Subject: Home

Hi, everyone,

I had the procedure this morning. It went well. A bit more involved than expected. I was fully sedated and have a catheter installed in my side so that I can drain, or I can go back in if needed. Yucky. I guess a nurse is coming out to educate me and help.

My doctor said there is a chance it won't happen again. If that is the case, they will remove the catheter.

Anyway, I am a little sorer now than expected because of a few pokey holes and stitches. The belly is down, not quite as far as I hoped, but I feel much lighter and do not feel the back strain.

I have my little station set up and will be resting for the rest of the day/night. Pizza delivery tonight. The kids will be happy. Hope to hit the garden tomorrow. Love you all.

Stacey

Sent: Wednesday, May 02, 2012
Subject: Not a good day

Hi, Mom,

I am not having a good morning. First of all, I don't notice much difference in my belly. I think it needs to be drained again. Secondly, I am in twice as much pain as yesterday. Mostly from the procedure.

I have this bandage mess on me, and I have no clue as to what to do or how to work this thing. I guess I am supposed to call some home nurse or something. I don't remember. I have a bunch of papers I am supposed to fax in to get the supplies. Confusing.

I will be seeing my doctor and nurses this a.m. Hopefully they will take care of me and get things back on track. The hospital was going to have a nurse call today, too. I am sure they will be helpful.

I just feel frustrated and in a quandary now. That's all. Hopefully something good will happen to brighten the day.

Stacey

Sent: Thursday, May 03, 2012
Subject: Good morning

Hi, Mom,

It looks like it is going to be a lovely day, between thunderstorms at least. I will plan to be outside or on the porch for part of it. I have someone coming to turn the other half of the veggie garden this afternoon. I might weed the edges (sitting down) and visit while he does that.

I have to be careful because I am leaking! I went to the ER last night, and everything checked out fine. I just need to heal a little more. They changed my bandages because I did not have any at home. I am going to write a letter and try to get my $150 co-pay back because I should have been provided with training and bandages sooner. For now, I am wearing a towel on my belly. That is how bad it is. The nurse is coming this a.m. I am hoping we can relieve some more fluid and pressure, although I consider what I lost last night a bonus!

Love Stacey

Sent: Friday, May 04, 2012
Subject: Camp and stuff

Hello,

Hope you had a good garage sale. If you had the same weather as us, you had a great day for it.

I went into the doc today just to make sure all was well. Things seemed pretty good. I did get fluids and magnesium. He also alleviated many concerns I had about this catheter and told me he was on call this weekend if I had any problems. That should keep me out of the ER. I will go into the center at the hospital on Monday to possibly have another extraction.

They agreed that it would be best not to do it at home for now.

I am trying to take it easy. I need to stay off my feet as much as possible this weekend. I hope to send the girls off on the walk tomorrow. I think they are excited.

I enjoyed some sunshine this afternoon and got a couple things done. One big thing was that I signed the kids up for camp. I faxed in the registration because when I called there was only one spot left in Kassia's group. Laurie, we signed up for the week of July 8th if you are interested in sending Remington.

Have a good weekend! Stacey

Sent: Wednesday, May 09, 2012
Subject: Hello

Hi, Mom,

Thanks for the generous gift! It will come in handy because guess who went to the ER again last night?

I was making dinner, and this catheter started leaking profusely. I have a couple of funny stories to share about that drama. I will wait until I see you.

Anyway, it was a pretty good day. I feel better. No fever or sore throat. Had chemo as planned.

Bloodwork good except magnesium low.

Cytology report on abdominal fluid was negative. :) Doc said this is good but not an absolute guarantee that nothing is going on in there.

He is still thinking about ablation but wants to find the right window.

Chemo plan will stay the same, but he may change the Erbitux to something else soon.

I got drained, and some more stitches were added to prevent leakage.

Right now, it looks like I may be going in three times per week for drainage. It goes very fast, and they are so super nice at that place. It is also ten minutes from home.

I am sore and achy from the big day. I will be resting tonight. Hoping we achieve a balance here within the next few days.

I will talk to you soon about the weekend. I don't think I should stray far from Elgin yet, but there is hope I will feel better and be able to get around more.

This is the third time in the last two weeks I found myself driving home in my pajamas. I hesitate, thinking I should run into the grocery store and get this or that. I am not quite that brave.

I am beginning to take humor in what has been a cruddy week. I am accumulating some good stories about body fluids, getting around Elgin in my pajamas, and have a couple of funny related Kobyisms.

My stretchy Old Navy clothes came today. We will see how those work out. Talk to you soon.

Love Stacey

Sent: Friday, May 11, 2012
Subject: Re: Hi

We had a very nice day, too. I did the dog walk and later soaked up some sunshine and read outside.

I developed another fever. No ER, thank goodness, but I was put on another antibiotic. We will see what the doc says. A little worried about infection at catheter site. I am also getting a cough, so it might be from what I had earlier in the week. I need to stay close to Elgin this weekend.

I would welcome your company and the extra hands. I just might be a little lazy. Looking forward to the *Desperate Housewives* finale on Sunday.

Stacey

Sent: Monday, May 14, 2012
Subject: Home

Hi,

It sounds you had a day of delays, too! Thank you for staying with me as long as you did. I sure did enjoy your company.

I had no idea I would be there so long. They set me loose at 2 p.m. Actually, I sort of walked out on my own. It bordered on the ridiculous, like I had nothing else to do but lay there all day. I think I will be ready to take care of this myself soon. The nurse today just got back from a conference and attended panels on these catheter things. The idea is to encourage lifestyle independence and activity (as opposed to being bedridden in a hospital room 12 hours per week!). They had patient speakers who said they do it on airplane flights, etc. I guess they are very common with ovarian cancer patients.

I got magnesium, and then they called the catheter doctor up to do stitches. I was grateful that she was willing to come to me instead of me go down to another part of the hospital.

Chocolates and potato salad to the rescue. It was good to come home to a fridge of leftovers. I loaded up a plate and sat outside and ate when I got home.

A pretty busy normal week in store. Band concerts, dentist appointments. I think I am ready to step back into it with caution. I love you, and thanks again for the visit and all the wonderful help.

Stacey

Sent: Wednesday, May 16, 2012
Subject: Hi

Hi, Mom,

I was pretty sick on Tuesday. I did manage to get down and videotape my speech, though. I had some pain in my lower back, left side, and threw up. I wasn't able to eat.

I called Dr. Y., and he sent me in to be drained again. This provided some relief.

I went home to bed and felt better at about 8 p.m. I am up now. I took a little pain medicine for my back because I started not sleeping well. Could be the kidney? I see my doctor early tomorrow. Will try to find out what is going on. May need some help soon if this keeps up.

Love Stacey

Sent: Friday, May 18, 2012
Subject: New drug

Dr. N., who works with Dr. Y., told me today there is a new drug set to come out in August. It sounds promising.

Feeling good after getting my fluids in/fluids out today. I planted half a flat of impatiens, did some much-needed watering, and picked about a pint of strawberries. Resting now. Tommy is making pizza. He said his meeting went very well today. What a nice day.

Love Stacey

Sent: Sunday, May 20, 2012

A pretty good day today. The nurse came out both today and yesterday and did the draining at home without incident. I will try next!

Early morning dog walk. A short one but nice.

We went to church. That was nice because I don't think I have been there for about a month.

Later I bought some mulch. I put down five bags. Tommy was away, so I actually was hauling the bags around. I wore myself out, but it felt good. I left some for when you come. :)

We did not get much rain. It was enough to wet the plants, so I did not feel bad about skipping a watering this evening.

Busy day of appointments starting at 8:30 tomorrow. I am hoping to be able to keep my massage and Dr. Jaena appointment. I am looking forward to those. Can't wait to see you.

Love Stacey

Sent: Friday, May 25, 2012
Subject: Hi

Thanks for the pics. It is good to see you made it home. I got a call at 2:30. They found my magnesium quite low. I had a choice to go in immediately or wait until Tuesday. So here I am until 5:30. Tommy will be home at 3:30 to greet the guests. This should help me feel better for the rest of the weekend.

Love, Stacey

Sent: Saturday, May 26, 2012
Subject: Re: Hi

A little more tired than I had hoped for but OK. I rested a lot. The kids had fun. Laurie helped finish off the laundry (folding socks) and such. Between you and her, it is all done! I can't remember the last time that happened.

I did my draining by myself this a.m. It went pretty smooth. That felt like a big accomplishment. Tommy was my backup assistant.

I garnered up some energy this afternoon and finished planting my garden. Laurie dug and planted the potatoes. It will be a very full garden. I need to run the sprinkler for a good hour or so now. She did some more watering for me. I will get out this evening and finish up. I have a feeling the next two days will be lazy inside days with the heat. We grilled out and got our sun today. We did not have thunder or rain last night. It is getting pretty serious with this drought. Have a good weekend.

Love Stacey

In May 2012, Stacey wrote a speech for Fox Valley Volunteer Hospice about her life after the cancer diagnosis and her experience with their services. A video of her speech was shown at their annual garden party with her in attendance.

Hi, Mom,

Here it is. I am hoping I can view the video on Tuesday. I may just go with that since everyone has worked so hard on it. A pretty good day today. Very lazy. I got out in the garden early this morning.

Love Stacey

Hello. It is an honor to be able to share my story with you today. My name is Stacey Reynolds. I am a mother of three beautiful children, a wife, a daughter, an interior designer, an environmentalist, a crazy gardener, a lifelong learner, a martial artist, and an artist with a paintbrush. If you were to see me on the street, you may peg me as a typical Volvo-driving soccer mom. What you would not realize is that I am a cancer survivor. I live with a diagnosis of advanced colon cancer each and every day.

I am not exactly a poster child for colon cancer. At the time of my diagnosis, I was 45 years old. Before my diagnosis, I was perceived to be in excellent health. I walked 1 to 2 miles per day, attended martial arts classes three days per week. I reached a lifelong goal of achieving my black belt rank just eight weeks before my diagnosis. I am a vegetarian, a conscious consumer who seeks out things that are green, organic, and non-toxic. I do not smoke, and there is no history of colon cancer in my family.

My age, good health, and lack of family history are the reasons why a colonoscopy was not ordered when I started having minor symptoms back in 2009, nine months before my official diagnosis. The symptoms I was having were easily attributed to something far more benign. It is my hope that each of you here today will take at least one important thing from my message. If you have any questionable symptoms, rule out the worst-case scenario first and GET SCREENED. For those of you that don't know, routine screening for colon cancer begins at age 50. On this journey, I have met many individuals younger than 50 who were in the same boat as me. Today I hope there are healthcare professionals out there who will hear me and will consider expanding their criteria for screening recommendations. For the rest of us, if you, a family member, or friend has symptoms, please GET SCREENED. There are all kinds of jokes and misperceptions about the colonoscopy procedure, but believe me—the procedure is a cake walk compared to extensive cancer treatment, and early detection improves survival rates substantially.

What I would like to talk to you about today is how I chose to LIVE my life after that big diagnosis in January 2010.

I can still hear that first doctor saying, "There is no cure for your stage of cancer. We can control it with chemotherapy much like a chronic illness." "I have seen others count their lives in months and some count their lives in years." As I leaned closer to my husband who was diligently taking notes, my thoughts flashed to our children, ages, 7, 9, and 11.

I closed my eyes and thought, "Three years. Just give me three years." I had so much more that I wanted to teach them and share with them. Today I stand here well on my way to that three-year mark, and I think I may have short-changed myself a little—or a lot.

The weeks ahead were a blur. There were many important decisions to be made. I have nothing but thanks for my husband, Tom, who attended each of those initial appointments with me and acted as my pillar of strength. This was not easy for him either. Together we figured it out, and I was pleased to find a local team of doctors that I was comfortable with and, to this date, have nothing but the highest praise for. In addition to traditional treatment, I sought out alternative therapies, such as acupuncture, reiki, and nutritional supplementation. I reduced my stress with yoga classes, meditation, and yes—gardening.

Just 12 days after diagnosis, I began my chemo treatment. I think my questions were the same as anyone else starting on this journey. Was I going to lose my hair? Would I be able to enjoy food again? How many of my normal activities am I going to be able to keep up with?

One of the first things I did was order a wig from the ACS website. It was a cute little red pixie cut. I also added several sweatshirts to my wardrobe. I guess I was thinking I just needed to be very comfortable. Each and every time I ate one of my favorite foods, I wondered whether it would be the last time I enjoyed it (I am a big fan of Thai and Mexican food).

I was wrong about a lot of things. First of all, my hair did not all fall out. The cute little wig sits on the shelf to this day. I occasionally wear sweatshirts, but I do find that I do get out of the house a lot, and I have a pretty versatile wardrobe to support my activities. Lastly, I still enjoy Thai and Mexican food. There are some days when it tastes better than others, but I still enjoy my food (chocolate and carrot cake are a couple of my other weaknesses).

The biggest surprise for me is how much I have been able to get out and enjoy a normal life. I am living each day with this cancer. My life was changed significantly with this diagnosis, but it hasn't been ALL bad. I cringe a little when I hear people say that having cancer is a battle, or so-and-so lost their battle to cancer. We all have our battles. They come in many shapes and forms. Nearly everyone I know is living with some form of battle.

I have been blessed with a good quality of life these past 28 months. I can truly say that my life has been rich, and I have learned more about living in these past two years than I have in the other 45 combined. Since my diagnosis, I have seen many milestones in my children's lives (proud mama moments is what I call them—I love my children dearly). I've seen the seasons come and go and enjoyed endless hours in my garden. I have watched sunsets over the ocean, ziplined through the rainforest, traveled to three different countries, creating memories with my family along the way. I've tried new recipes, read many books, redecorated our house, shared romantic outings with my husband, and have enjoyed several holidays with my large, loving family. I've been able to teach my kids more about life, perhaps in a more meaningful way than ever before. Most of all, I have seen the beauty in others. I have so much gratitude for the extended family, friends, neighbors, and church members who have reached out to me and my family. I've learned about love and how it surrounds us everywhere. I have so much gratitude for all of it.

I realize that not everyone is dealt the same cards when it comes to cancer treatment. Everyone reacts to therapies differently and has their own set of circumstances and makes their own decisions on which paths to follow. Some will say that attitude is everything. I think that there is some truth to this.

I do not know what the future holds for me (none of us do really), but I will share eight of my strategies that have helped me on this journey. Perhaps it will help some of you living while dealing with your own battles.

1. Shed fears: What are you afraid of? Write it down. Confront fears (Harry Potter reference).

2. Take care of yourself. Make time for yourself. Diet.

3. Enjoy the present. Every day is different.

4. Stay connected.

5. Take pleasure in the small things.

6. Seek out new experiences.

7. Never stop dreaming.

8. Accept help. Hmm... this was probably one of the hardest things for me. It was almost exactly a year ago that I first contacted Fox Valley Volunteer Hospice. I had received a brochure from a friend sometime after my diagnosis. It took me a while to call. I will have to admit that the word *hospice* scared me. I sure did not think I was ready for any hospice care—after all, I was still attending martial arts classes and could do 30 push-ups, I was taking care of a household, volunteering in community organizations, and helping in my children's schools.

In spite of this, I realized that something was missing. I had so much support surrounding me and my family already, but there was a hole, and this hole had left me with some unease that was getting in the way of my "living." I knew my health could take a turn for the worse at any time, and when this happened the cards would begin to fall. What I felt like me and my family needed was a H-U-G-E safety net that we could fall into, should this happen. I thought about my children and their need to be plugged in. I wanted to make sure they felt they had someone to turn to, to share any fear or concerns they had now or in the future.

I gave FVVH a call and inquired about their We Care services. With my life-threatening illness, I seemed to fit the criteria for the type of person they were reaching out to. I spoke to Janine and set up an appointment to meet. Our initial meeting went well (she is a very kind and warm person). Afterwards, I felt this immense sense of ease. I signed the paperwork, and it seemed a huge load was lifted—a final piece to a puzzle had been found. THIS MEANT THE WORLD TO ME—IT FREED ME SO THAT I COULD LIVE.

As time went on, I found that the services provided through We Care were much more than a safety net. I have my personal volunteers who meet with me weekly to listen to my physical, emotional, and spiritual needs. In reality, many weeks are spent listening to how I have "lived" the past week. Most importantly, these volunteers see me where I am at each week, and believe me, it can be a roller-coaster ride from one week to the next. I have been so impressed with the professionalism and dedication of these volunteers who give so much of themselves to be there for me.

The other staff members and professionals who have worked with me and the rest of my family have also impressed me with their excellence and dedication. They have worked with my family for almost a year now. I have seen the changes in my children. Each of them expresses it in a different way, but I perceive it as a sense of relief and comfort they did not have before.

Janine and Christy have been there for me to listen to all the good and bad twists in my diagnosis and treatment, ready to offer support and referrals wherever needed. They've come to my home, they've visited me in the hospital, and have remained a phone call away should any questions or concerns arise.

My thanks go out to Janine, Christy, Sandy, Arturo, Donna, Paula, Merit, and all the others working behind the scenes. You should be very proud of your organization and all the differences you are making in people's lives. I think that the name We Care says it all. You have exceeded my expectations, and I am forever grateful for all that you do.

CHAPTER 26

Darling Stacey Is the Most Awesome Person in the World

Sent: Friday, June 01, 2012
Subject: Pretty flowers

Here is a picture of my lovely flowers. The pretty roses and sunflowers are from you. I was lucky to win the centerpiece at the garden party at my table and got to bring the geraniums home. Now where to plant them…. Thanks. A moderately better day today.

Love Stacey

Sent: Friday, June 01, 2012
Subject: Re: Pretty flowers

There were many good things about the day but too much hustle and bustle. First got to rest just about the time the kids came home— and they were wound up. Last full day.

I think the morning was rough because the maids came at 9 a.m., and the dog and I had to be out of the way. I really need an hour to rest after the draining and shouldn't schedule anything before 10. I can't complain, though. I went out and had a nice breakfast while the house was being cleaned. :) I had to catch up on some e-mails and calls I have neglected. One of them was approval for the rain garden—deadline yesterday.

I also felt like I needed to talk to my doctor. I was SO disappointed when he wasn't in yesterday. Nothing really new. He wasn't overly alarmed about anything but thinks it is the liver enlarging causing pressure. I don't think any of my counts are horrible, but my bilirubin may be a little elevated. Need sunshine, which won't be hard to find. Spent two hours waiting for a five-minute visit.

Looking forward to seeing Lesley. The flowers were cheery.

Love Stacey

Sent: Monday, June 04, 2012
Subject: Hospital

I am being admitted tonight for a couple of days.

Doc is concerned about leg swelling. One of my liver counts that has never been high went way up. Pretty serious. White counts are extremely high. Hemoglobin is really low. No transfusion yet.

Hopefully we can get it all leveled off and I will feel better. I will keep you posted. Tell me if you want to come.

Love Stacey

I didn't realize it until much later, but this is probably the kindest letter I have ever received. Tommy was telling us in the gentlest of ways that Stacey was dying. He had warned her doctors in the beginning to never tell her anything that would cause her to lose hope. The letter left room for us to have hope as well.

From: Thomas Lesiewicz
Date: Wed, 13 Jun 2012
Subject: darling Stacey is the most awesome person in the world

Hi, Guys,

First, I wanted to say thank you for all the time you have been spending at our house helping out. We can all see how much her condition has changed over the last month.

Stacey and I haven't had a lot of time to just talk about things recently, but I spoke to her this morning, and she is hoping her recent downturn is because of the current cocktail of chemo drugs she is on. That is good. She is hopeful. We all know she is a fighter!!! So, I wanted to share that with everyone.

We never know what the future brings. There can be a cure for cancer tomorrow—we just don't know.

I think I mentioned it to people individually when they were at the house, but things are kind of a blur, so I just wanted to reiterate it. We don't know what tomorrow brings, but what I do know is that I feel it is my job to make sure she can spend as much time with family and friends as humanly possible. Knowing Stacey, I think that is the most important thing. I know the accommodations are not the greatest, but you guys (anyone else) have an open invitation to stay and or visit anytime. Don't feel all doom and gloom, and don't feel like you have to. Just know that if you want to visit anytime, you can. Just like Stacey has a permanent "get out of jail free" card, you guys have a permanent "come and visit anytime you want" invitation.

Second, don't feel like you "have" to do chores, unless Stacey asks you to. Then of course her wishes over-ride anything I say. ;) I know keeping myself busy is sometimes helpful in keeping my mind at ease, and sometimes it gives me a good feeling knowing I am doing something tangible for someone else. I realize other people probably feel the same way. Just know you shouldn't feel compelled to do things like that. Sometimes just keeping the kids from bothering her too much is good enough so she can get her nap time in. There are also tons of neighbors and friends who keep asking me, "What can I do? Call me if there is anything I can do," and it is a testament to Stacey that she has so many people who love her and are willing to help out.

Third, I think you all have it but in case you don't, my cell number is below.

Stacey can be a little hard to reach sometimes, and with the phone ringing off the hook, it sometimes disturbs her naps. If you can't reach Stacey, then please by all means, call me. You can call anytime. You can ask me any questions you want. There are no awkward questions; there is nothing wrong you can say. It is just good for us to communicate, and I wanted to let you know it is OK to call me anytime. You can also share my number with anyone you want. Same ground rules. Anyone can call me anytime they want. For any reason. Family, friends, whatever.

Again, in closing, I don't want to be all doom and gloom.

Stacey is hopeful and knowing how tough she is... she will probably be alive and kicking 25 years from now. But today is the best day of my life because Stacey is alive today! I just want you to know (and spread the word) that if you want to maximize your Stacey-time, then that's cool. It is all about Stacey.

—tml—

On 6/13/2012 1:09 PM
Carole Young wrote:

Thanks, Tommy. I will be back! Hope to see you in a couple of days at Fay Lake. I can't express in words how grateful I am my little girl married a wonderful guy like you.

From: Thomas Lesiewicz
Sent: Wednesday, June 13, 2012
Subject: Re: darling Stacey is the most awesome person in the world

Hope to see you at Fay Lake!! I can't express in words how grateful I am you made your little girl so that I could marry her. ;)

Date: Thu, 14 Jun 2012
Subject: Hi

Hi, Mom and Gary,

Hope you are having a great time. Laurie and I had a nice visit. She was extremely helpful.

I am feeling pretty good. Still swollen, but mornings seem good. It creeps up by end of day. Got some slow-acting diuretics. I should enjoy myself if I can. Sit back and not overdo.

I e-mailed Fay Lake to ask about the stairs/bathroom issue (bedrooms up, bathroom down). They were very nice and may see if we can trade units with our neighbors. They have a sofa sleeper in that unit. Or they can bring one in. They said they could even use one of your trundles and move it.

I did find out our neighbors are only there for one night. I don't know which night. If you wanted to, you might inquire about it (if you were interested in the townhouse). It may also add confusion. It sounds like we could have one noisy night—a group of ATV riders.

We did rent an SUV—a Ford Expedition. It looks roomy and comfortable. Gotta keep the princess comfortable or she becomes a witch!

Love Stacey

From: Carole Young
Sent: Monday, June 18, 2012
Subject: Stacey

Hi, all,

Tommy e-mailed me that they got home from Fay Lake about 5:30 today and that the trip seemed to go better. But when they got home, Stacey called the home health nurse because her blood pressure was very low, and the nurse told her to go to the ER.

Tommy said she was "very, very weak." But Stacey said the trip was worth it, seeing family and all. Tommy said he was sure they would admit her to the hospital.

Mom/Carole

From: Stacey Reynolds
Sent: Thursday, June 21, 2012

My updates as of this morning:

Numbers were much better on labs. The sodium was the main concern. It is back to where it was three weeks ago.

They brought in a kidney specialist, not because they thought something was wrong with my kidneys but to take a look at the whole picture and try to balance the electrolytes. The kidney doctors have taken a couple of approaches. The first did not work, (pumped me with a lot of fluids to bring pressure up and then give electrolyte boosts with IV). The second seems to be working better. Limit fluids by mouth. One liter in per day, one liter out by drain. I have been taking a pill to raise blood pressure. I don't know if that will continue when I am out. It still is not very high. I have been off the IV and fluids since yesterday. That is nice.

Other than that, I feel better today. My legs seem a little less swollen. I was worried because last night I felt very weak. But today I feel stronger.

It sounds like I will be going home later. Missed all the hot weather, darn. Thank you for all the well wishes and help. Love you all.

Stacey

Sent: Saturday, June 23, 2012
Subject: Hi

Hi, Mom,

We look forward to your visit. I didn't mean to put a kibosh on your Brussel sprout idea. All along I have been saying I want to eat healthy, but too much prep involved. I would love help with this!

Kassia is cleaning her room so Lesley can sleep on the futon up there.

Love Stacey

From: Thomas Lesiewicz
Sent: Friday, June 29, 2012
Subject: Stacey is low on sodium

Hello, Everyone,

The results are in... nothing too radical/shocking/worrisome... she has low sodium. The doc said it is the lowest he has seen it for her and has likely been low for a few days (which is weird, because they just released her a few days ago). She will be here overnight. :(

The doc is the same one she has seen in the ER the last three times. So, he knows her history, and he has already spoken to her other doctors. He said they just need to come up with a long-term plan. :)

I'll update you as I know more. She is resting peacefully with a smile on her face awaiting a move from the ER to a regular room.

From: Thomas Lesiewicz
Sent: Tuesday, July 03, 2012, 1:46 PM
Subject: Stacey update

The nurse just called me with an update at 4 a.m. Her BP was the highest they have seen since she has been this time in the hospital (94). Her BP it is about 87 now (not bad, but not high enough to drain). Her sodium is about 123 (it has been holding at about 123–126 for the past day or so). They are limiting her intake of fluids because it is still building up and can't drain (because her BP is under 95). If they do drain, they'll have to do it in the ICU where they can do it safely if her BP drops too low. Her legs still have compression wraps on them (below the knee), and they have to stay on for one week. She got her head shaved yesterday (now she looks like me). We have an appointment at 6 p.m. to talk to what sounds like a promising hospice provider. They will do bloodwork, monitoring of magnesium, potassium, and sodium. With home health care nurses, they can get a hospital bed.

She will have her interventional radiologists checking in on her today to follow up on her drain leaking problem. I talked to Stacey this morning, and she sounded a little more with it.

She's been very sleepy and sleeping a lot. She's getting lots of positive energy from people doing reiki and other alternative healing (including Dr. Jaena). Not sure when she'll be home.

From: Thomas Lesiewicz
Sent: Tuesday, July 03, 2012 3:22 PM
Subject: Re: Stacey update

Positive energy is great.

Call her anytime you want—the room is best.

As for the rest of the week... right now I have no in-person appointments booked, so I can work from home Thursday and Friday. The unknowns are when Stacey is coming home, what type of care will she need, and what type of care will be available. I may know more about this after our 6 p.m. meeting at the hospital.

For the camp... when do they have to be there? Is there a certain time/date when they have to be there?

Carole

On Friday, July 6, Gary and I drove to Elgin for a visit and to pick up the kids to take them to Sugar Creek Bible Camp in Ferryville, Wisconsin. It is a camp that Stacey had, herself, attended as a child. When she registered them for camp in April, she felt fortunate to get all three of them enrolled in the same week in July. It is a very popular camp, and they would all be in different levels of camp life according to their age. Because she was able to accomplish this, they were not home at the time of her death.

Before we left for home on Saturday, Stacey suddenly became concerned about Kassia's food allergies and tried to make a list for her to take to camp. She was struggling but didn't seem distressed that what should have been a routine task was now difficult. Since I was familiar with the allergies, I took over and I listed them out loud as I wrote them down. She nodded after each one, and then mouthed, "and chick peas." She smiled and made a peace sign with her fingers as I took the last photograph she would appear in with her children.

Sunday was the day we drove from our home in Boscobel to deliver the kids to Sugar Creek in Ferryville. It was hot, and the registration lines were long. The line for special medical issues because of Kassia's food allergies was especially long. The kids were happy when they were able to join their fellow campers in their individual locations, and Grandpa and Grandma were happy to head for home.

That evening I drove back to Elgin with daughter Laurie and granddaughter Remington. Laurie had talked to Tommy on the phone earlier, and we were both worried that the news about her sister was not good. The three of us spent the night at their house. The next day, July 9, was Laurie's birthday.

CHAPTER 27
Carole's Story

There is a belief held by some and expressed by Robert Swartz in his book, *Your Soul's Plan: Discovering the Real Meaning of the Life You Planned Before You Were Born*, that your soul is instrumental in planning certain aspects of your life in advance of your birth. The process involves predestination with an element of free will thrown in.

My daughter Stacey died July 9, 2012, on her younger sister Lauren's birthday. If it is possible for people to choose their time to leave this earth, why would anyone choose to die on a loved-one's special day? As it turns out, we will be reminded every July 9th there are life events to celebrate as we remember with sadness that was the day she left us.

From the experience, at the same time that I question the fairness of it all and go through all the "whys" and "if onlys," I am more aware that life's journey presents us with lessons to be learned and mini miracles to experience if one remains open and receptive. "Miracles surround us at every turn, if we but sharpen our perceptions to them."—Willa Cather

Stacey's husband, Tommy, found her memorial service outline among her papers after she died. She requested the tone of the service be: "Don't cry because it's over; smile because it happened"—Dr. Seuss.

• • •

I am sitting on the big leather hassock in the living room looking out the doggy nose-smeared window at the small yellow bungalow across the street, watching Sonia. She is blowing grass off the sidewalk with a leaf blower. Every day she emerges from that house with a smoothie for Stacey. They are large smoothies and have started piling up in the refrigerator because she can't drink them as fast as they keep coming. Once it was a black bean and rice casserole for the family. It went uneaten. No one has much of an appetite, and the Hispanic dish was unfamiliar to picky kids. I could tell it was probably delicious, but I had to throw it out and wash the dish so I could give it back to her. Her gifts of food come from her heart and are always offered with tears and words of how hard she is praying.

There are two men from the Unitarian Church here building stair railings to make it easier for her to go up the short landing into the kitchen and up the stairs to the bedroom. That it's too late for that doesn't matter. They work with concentrated energy, ignoring everything else going on. The care and craftsmanship put into the beautifully carved and sanded wooden railings would be appreciated and admired by her if she was in any shape to notice them. It is a gift they can give. That is all that matters.

Two days ago, when her stepdad and I left to take the grandkids to Sugar Creek Bible Camp, we dropped off a rather large volume book at the library. I asked first if she wanted it renewed or returned. It was a hopeful question but we both really knew the answer. And, she said, there was another book, a Native American Book. She thought it, too, had come from the library. I found a small book on the shelf in the living room, *Keep Going* by Joseph M. Marshall III. It had a picture of a Buffalo on the cover. "Native American, for sure," I thought. She acknowledged that was the book, but there was no indication it was a library book, so I put it back on the shelf.

I am back in Elgin now, and she is in a hospital bed that was delivered to the house while I was gone. The bed takes up most of the room in the small office at the front of the house. "The Water Room," she calls it, and she has decorated it with all things about water. There are pictures of the kids at Fay and Lost Lakes, a grandmother's oval picture of an old mill with water wheel, and an oil painting of a child with a watering can that had hung in her other grandmother's house. When Grandma Agnes died, we found a small note on the back that said, "Give this to Stacey when I am gone."

There is an eclectic bunch of people in the house today—family, friends, her holistic doctor, Dr. Jaena, the reiki therapist, her Bible study group of neighbor women, and Sandy, her hospice friend. Husband Tommy's tall presence hovers over it all, as he paces from room to room making sure all of her last wishes are met: keep the noise level down, quiet reading to her of passages from *Walden*, no lingering hand-holding (too confining, she had said), and no last-minute efforts to "save her soul."

Although she knew the truth of what she was facing and had been preparing for it, her contact with me was always honest but upbeat and hopeful. That she had written a "memorial service outline" revealed the truth that she kindly hid from me, throughout the illness.

I enter the water room quietly. She lies very still in the hospital bed with eyes closed. Her every breath is an effort. I want to breathe for her. The disease has progressed quickly over the last couple of weeks, dealing cruelly with the familiar beauty of her face and body. She has gone all two and a half years after the diagnosis without losing her hair until very recently. I ask Tommy for the head scarf she had been wearing the day we left with the grandkids. "It might be a little wet," he said. Someone has washed it. I arrange it as attractively as I can around her head and then used a damp washcloth to wash the corners of her mouth. I say to her, "It's been a long time since I have washed your face."

A well-meaning friend peeks in the French doors of the office and offers a rather blunt comment. "She can hear you," I admonish. I am not sure it's true.

I hold her hand a little bit, but not too much. I tell her Jesus loves her, but I know I don't need to save her soul.

I don't read from *Walden*. Instead I get the book, *Keep Going*, by Joseph M. Marshall III off the bookshelf and randomly start reading a passage.

> Grandfather says this: "Being strong means taking one more step toward the top of the hill, no matter how weary you may be. It means letting the tears flow through the grief. It means to keep looking for the answer, though the darkness of despair is all around you. Being strong means to cling to hope for one more heartbeat, one more sunrise. Each step, no matter how difficult, is one more step closer to the top of the hill. To keep hope alive for one more heartbeat at a time leads to the light of the next sunrise, and the promise of a new day."
> (Joseph M. Marshall. 2009. *Keep Going: The Art of Perserverance.* New York: Sterling Ethos. 125.)

My voice breaks as I read it, and the tears start flowing as well. I look over at her and see a tear slowly edging down *her* cheek. I was right. She can hear me.

When my siblings and I sang our 94-year-old mother over into the next world with hymns remembered from childhood, the nurses at Good Samaritan nursing home opened the window to the cold February day wide enough for her soul to escape. It was their tradition.

In contrast, it is a hot and humid summer day when Stacey leaves us. My thoughts take me back to that winter day and Good Samaritan nursing home. The window in the water room is already open. Someone earlier placed a vase of garden flowers on the sill, and a breeze moves the lace curtains slightly. On the other side of the window is her natural prairie rain garden. I walk out through the living room where everyone, stunned, is mourning in their own way. Through the kitchen I go and out the back door, around the house to the rain garden. I am still thinking about souls and where they go once they escape the rooms of houses, out through windows. Every part of me wants it to be true. I look up as I think, "Up, a soul would go up." Above me, in the sky, is a lone white cloud, with an opening in the shape of a heart, a perfect cookie cutter shaped heart. A feeling of peace and wonder entered my soul that day standing alone in my daughter's rain garden and has remained with me ever since.

Three days later, we are home again in Wisconsin. A memorial service has been planned for August 8, next month, Stacey's birthday, at the Unitarian Church in Elgin. In an attempt to get back into my old morning routine, I settle down on the couch with a cup of coffee in front of *Good Morning America* with the puzzle page of the *Wisconsin State Journal* on my lap desk and began to decode the Cryptoquote. The solution that morning: "Don't cry because it's over; smile because it happened."—Dr. Seuss.

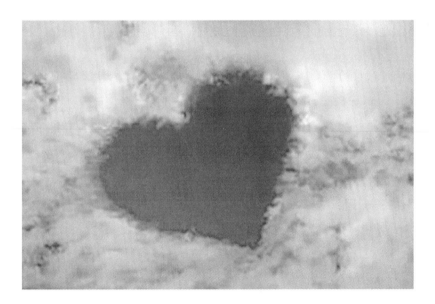

CHAPTER 28
Memorial Service

Memorial Service Outline
Stacey Reynolds
Prepared on February 2, 2012, Happy Groundhog Day!

My wish is to be cremated.

I would like to have my ashes buried/scattered. I would like to have some ashes scattered or buried with two young or newly planted trees, preferably oak. I have an affinity for oak trees and the strength that they represent. One tree would be in Elgin, the other tree would be in Boscobel, Wisconsin. I would like the remaining ashes to be set free in the Wisconsin River in the open area east of the Boscobel bridge. This would represent bringing me back to my childhood home. It is also a new beginning full of unlimited possibilities. The Wisconsin flows into the Mississippi, which flows into the Gulf of Mexico, etc. I also consider this area extremely beautiful (the bluffs, eagles, Easter Rock, and the trees).

I have an urn which I would like my ashes to be stored in temporarily—until they are ready to be set free. I purchased an antique Moroccan urn for my 40th birthday. It is a beautiful urn, and I feel it has an interesting story or past life. I remember purchasing it at a neighborhood antique store for $60 and bringing it home in the red wagon. I later found that it was valued at over $1,000. Besides it being a great deal and nice-looking, there was a reason why I purchased it that day, which is clear to me now. I've admired this urn for seven years now and would like to be part of its story.

The Service:

Event and tone: Don't be sad that it's over, be happy that it happened—Dr. Seuss

Be present, experience each day like it is your last, and plant some good seeds close to home. I have been a doer for my entire life. I considered myself very energetic and always had several projects on my plate. Over the past two years, I have learned a lot about life. I have learned that it is not about the lists, the doing, the accomplishments, or the travels. Instead it is the sunrises and sunsets, the laughter and smiles of children, love, seeing the beauty and goodness in those around me, and the millions of miracles that surround us every day. I've lived with a perceived "death sentence" for over two years now. For me, it felt more like a wake-up call, a call to start living. As odd as it sounds, I feel blessed to have had a chance to experience this. I would wish this for everyone (without the cancer part!).

When I look back on my life, I think that my most important accomplishments did not come from my career (yes, I did have one!). I am happy with my life, and if I could do it again, I would only plant more gardens! My most important works were the seeds that I planted close to home. The time I spent with my family, with my children, their schools, my church, in my neighborhood community, in my larger Elgin community working on sustainability projects. Though small in the grand scheme of things, these activities completed me. I am hoping that I served as a catalyst and that someday some of my seeds will flourish.

Personal Statement of Spiritual Belief:

I believe in a magnificent force or love that connects the universe. It has been accessible to me at all times. I am most likely to experience it by observing the miracles in nature or looking into the eyes of other people. I believe that this love or force will journey with my soul to the other side perhaps in a more profound way.

Of course, if I am wrong... I am OK with that too. I have had a wonderful life in this realm, and if this is all there is, I think that I will make very good compost with all of the green juice I have been drinking over the past couple of years.

Readings:

I have selected some short readings from Thoreau as possible readings. If I was to pick a book that had the most influence on my life, it would be *Walden* by Henry David Thoreau. I read this book while vacationing in New Orleans with Tommy. It seemed an unlikely place to explore transcendentalism. The mix of jazz and Cajun music and the clubs on Bourbon Street were intoxicating, to say the least. It must have been the right mix because something profound happened on this trip. I made decisions that guided the way I lived the rest of my adult life. After this trip, I lived with more awareness and intention. The principles in *Walden* shaped my design career, and from that point on, I considered myself a "green designer." I carefully researched the impacts that go into our building material choices—a deeper form of design that went beyond aesthetics. Eventually I was lucky to land a job where I could teach and guide others (this was in the early '90s before green design was in vogue).

Music:

"Ripple" by the Grateful Dead from *American Beauty*. I like the lyrics and think it is one of the most beautiful songs out there. The song has some spiritual qualities that ring true for me. I also do not know if many people know I am a closet Deadhead.

Instead of flowers:

I would like to have everyone that attends the service go out and plant something big or small afterwards. Depending on the season, seeds, seedlings, or plant starts could be provided. If this is impossible due to season or other limitations, I would suggest that they donate to Elgin Community Garden Network or Living Lands and Water, Million Tree Project. My family would enjoy hearing about what everyone plants or donates afterwards.

Dear extended family,

I am very sad to send the news that our daughter Stacey passed away yesterday at her home after a long battle with cancer. Such a brave and beautiful person. I am very proud of the way she lived and in awe of how she protected us and prepared us for her death. She was not in pain. She was at peace. She leaves her wonderful husband, Tommy, and three children, Aleks, 13; Kassia, 11; and Jakoby, 9. There will be a memorial service at their church later this month. Not sure of the exact date yet.

If you are on Facebook, please don't post until Tommy has a chance to announce it on Stacey's page.

Carole

The Reverend Dan Brosier, minister of The Unitarian Universalist Church of Elgin, and friend and neighbor of Stacey and Tommy officiated at Stacey's memorial and shared his "memories of Stacey." Sister, Laurie; brother, Garret; and stepdad, Gary read the *Walden* quotes.

The sanctuary was filled that evening so that some people had to take seats in an outer room. Parking went beyond space in the parking lot, and volunteers helped to direct cars to space in an adjacent field.

Rev. Dan Brosier—Early on, I heard that Stacey was having a colonoscopy. "No big deal," I said to myself. "Happens all the time. The procedure is uncomfortable, but routine." They couldn't find anything wrong, I was sure, or if they did it would be something so minor that they could treat it easily. Later, I heard there were going to be more tests. Again, "nothing to worry about," I said to Stacey and Tom. "A minor complication perhaps, nothing the doctors can't fix." Stacey and Tom looked at each other. In their eyes there was more concern than there was before.

I told myself that it had to be okay. After all, this is Stacey, vegetarian Stacey, no toxic chemicals Stacey, organic food Stacey, black belt Stacey, active and involved Stacey. What was she? Maybe 42? 43?... 46, years old. Young!

Then the diagnosis came back... and she stood right there, where she is sitting now, in front of us, and lit a candle and told us the news, and everyone was shocked. Many of us were in denial. It can't be, it can't be. It just can't be.

Look at her. She looks great! I saw her walking the family dog, Midnight. They both moved at a healthy pace. She was out working in the garden the other day, and when I talk with her, she sounds like the Stacey before the illness.

Then there were the tests that showed maybe they might have stopped the growth of the tumors. Maybe that new drug coming out will even be more effective. Maybe she's beating it. "Please keep her safe from the disease. Keep the disease at bay! Please let her stay in our lives. It is NOT HER TIME." But, it was.

Maybe there is an afterlife where we will see Stacey again, or maybe there is a spirit that survives the physical self, and Stacey's spirit will stay with us at our side whispering her gentle guidance and support throughout the years. There are all sorts of ideas about what happens after death. What I know for sure is that death is not the end of our relationship with Stacey.

Stacey lives on in each of us who knew her. In times spent with her, she is woven into the fabric of our lives and will remain there throughout our years influencing and shaping the unfolding of our lives.

I'm more aware of environmental issues because of Stacey. I've started a patch of garden in the easement in front of my house. These little gardens will forever in my mind be known as "Stacey Gardens" since hers was the first one I saw.

I'm more cautious about the potential harm of chemicals in our home because of Stacey. We tested for radon in our basement because of Stacey.

I have more faith in the power of citizenship involvement thanks to Stacey.

I understand better that one does not have to yell to be heard. That a soft and determined voice can bring about change and can be heard just as well as those who yell. And whenever I look upon the Labyrinth, which is out back of the church I will remember Stacey. She and Aleks and Kassia and Koby spent countless hours weeding the Labyrinth throughout a couple of summers. She was not afraid to get her hands dirty.

Yes, I will remember Stacey for the rest of my life, I will carry memories of her and what she believed in because she is woven into my life, into all our lives. We keep her spirit alive through our memories and our work towards greater justice and environmental sustainability, which she cared about so much.

Yes, I will remember.

CHAPTER 29

I Have Found Another Spot

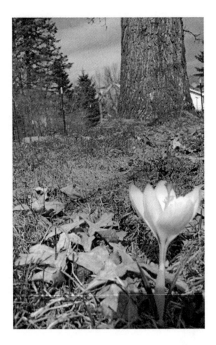

From: Lesley Reynolds
Sent: Sunday, April 28, 2013
Subject: Stacey flower

The very first flower I discovered blooming in our yard was in a very strange place—right in the middle of the lawn under the big oak tree. A spring hello? Maybe. Here are a few pictures of it. Lesley

From: Carole Young
Sent: Sunday, April 28, 2013
To: Lesley Reynolds
Subject: RE: Stacey flower

Of course.

From: Lesley Reynolds
Sent: Monday, May 13, 2013
To: Mom
Subject: one more thing

I had a Stacey dream last night. It was a really vivid one again. She looked healthy and vibrant and content, and she was with Grandma at the end of it. Whenever I have a dream like that, I wake up feeling at peace and not sad at all. It always seems like she was really there, and it feels like a gift to be able to see her again for a little bit. (I guess writing about it is making me a little sad now... but mostly it's a good thing.) Love, Lesley

Arrangements are made in the fall to distribute Stacey's ashes according to her wishes.

From: Carole Young
Sent: Friday, October 11,2013
To: Lesley Reynolds
Subject: RE: hi

Yes, I will be around. I will be making cookies and pies for the Lesiewicz family. Tommy says they will start out Sunday about 9:00. He said Stacey specified that the ashes should be done in the morning with the sun in the East, so he wants to do that Monday morning. Mom

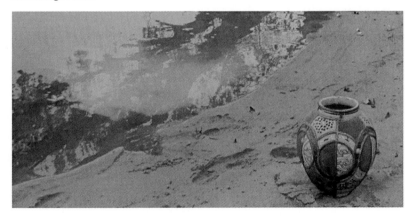

Carole

Morning haze blurs textures and fall colors and flattens the contours of the hills turning them into two-dimensional backdrops on the opposite side of the river.

We gather this October morning—her husband, children, mother and stepfather, brother and wife—in the place she specified. It is not an easy task, but it is what she asked of us.

The Moroccan urn sits in the sand at the edge of the lapping water. As Tommy removes the plastic bags of ashes from it and pours them slowly into the river, a fire siren from the city just south of us rips into the silence and seems to express to the universe what is in our hearts. This is not fair! This is too hard to bear!

The sun breaks through the haze, sharpening colors and the shapes of hills across the river as we pause there in silence before getting in our cars to leave. This place will forever now be a sacred place to us.

From: Lesley Reynolds
Sent: Monday, October 14, 2013
Subject: Stacey's fall flower
Attachments: IMG_2491 .JPG

I found this lone flower under the oak tree in our yard this morning. It's in the exact same place that first little flower peeped out of the snow in the spring.

The first and last flowers of the season. :)

From: Carole Young
Sent: Monday, October 14, 2013
To: Lesley Reynolds
Subject: RE: Stacey's fall flower

Beautiful little flower.

Tommy found the story Stacey was writing. He left it here because he said he had it on his hard drive. There are a few paragraphs about that place on the river:

"The morning sun glazes the water. The skies are clear. Beyond the river, an eagle soars above one of the bluffs. I stare into the swirling waters in front of me. I sit on one of the rocks and close my eyes and breathe deeply. It is good to be alive. It is good to be present in this spot right now. If I should die, it is here that I would like to be laid to rest, not in the cemetery."

From: Carole Young
Sent: Monday, October 14, 2013
To: Lesley
Subject: Today on the river
Attachments: ashes 024.JPG; ashes 023.JPG; ashes 022. JPG; ashes 021 .JPG

It was a foggy morning, but the sun was coming out by the time we put the ashes in the water.

CHAPTER 30
At Peace with My Own Mortality

Carole

In Stacey's memorial service outline, she requested she be cremated and her ashes be divided and buried under oak trees in Boscobel and Elgin and also placed into the waters of the Wisconsin River.

The family, when trying to find a suitable oak tree in Boscobel, decided that one on her sister Laurie's property in the country would be safe from city tree trimmers and removers.

Tommy had found the stories Stacey had been writing and brought them with him when he came in October to distribute her ashes. We were amazed after reading one of Stacey's stories in its entirety that she had picked that tree first.

From: Carole Young
Sent: Monday, October 14, 2013 11:41 AM
Subject: photos from Sun. & Mon.
Attachments: ashes 016.JPG; ashes 014.JPG; ashes 012.JPG

We put some of Stacey's ashes under an oak tree at the top of the hill at Laurie's house.

From: Carole Young
Date: Mon, 14 Oct 2013 12:23
Subject: Stacey's story

I think we picked the right oak tree (by accident?). I was reading the story Stacey wrote that Tommy left me.

From: Thomas Lesiewicz
Sent: Monday, October 14, 2013 4:28 PM
Subject: Re: Stacey's story

I don't think anything was by accident...

From: Carole Young
Sent: Monday, October 14, 2013 5:03 PM
To: Tommy
Subject: RE: Stacey's story

Tommy, I just read the whole story. It starts out with a memory of a visit to Fay Lake with family when she was a teenager, then continues with a future she imagines for your family. It is a great one with all of the kids successful in their careers, Wisconsin with a new governor, and the world a better place all together. (And you get a Harley!) Then a return to the present and reality where it seems she was looking for some special places. Places where we ended up the last few days. What a remarkable person. I am in awe! Hope you had a great trip home. Sure enjoyed the visit.

Love Carole

Stacey's Story

June 2011—It was 10 a.m., and I did the final sweep through the house before loading the kids into the car and heading off on our four-hour journey in southern Wisconsin. Earlier this morning, the window guys had come and were busy changing our storm windows over. I took a walk around the house and gave my nod of approval. A smile of satisfaction crossed my face as I looked at the shiny new windows from the outside. On the inside, I was even more thrilled to see that I can now gaze clearly out through my kitchen windows. I looked up. Even the crystal I had hung there was in need of cleaning to regain its sparkle. I grabbed the crystal and headed for the door.

The mood was jolly as we jumped on the freeway and headed off on our journey. We listened to our favorite CDs, singing along to the familiar tunes. Some of the songs were preschool favorites we have been listening to for years. The kids laughed as we sang "The Wheels on the Bus." We snacked our way across Northern Illinois.

Tickle-belly hills is what we call them—the rolling hills that greet our entry into the driftless region, a land untouched by glaciers, today a land of beauty and wonder, my land! We stopped for a picnic at a scenic spot just outside of Galena. Any illusions I had of a perfect picnic were shattered, first by the amount of snacks we had consumed in the last 150 miles and secondly by the gnats that were buzzing around freely. We nibbled on sandwiches and popped a few grapes into our mouths. For some reason, I was suddenly inspired to start bombing the kids with grapes. This they found humorous and quite surprising. I am loving my new-found spontaneity, which creeps in at the strangest moments these days. Next we ran and played tag on top of the hill. I nearly wet my pants after all of the water I just drank, but it felt fun. It felt good to be running. It felt good to be a child again. With the panorama unfolding in front of us, it seemed we could run for miles.

It was one of those trips where a 3.5-hour trip somehow turned into five hours. A little road construction here, a detour there, and then there are the bathroom stops. Finally we made it to my parents' house in Wisconsin.

It felt good to relax after the endless drive. When I got to my parents' house, I felt engulfed in a feeling of warmth. I surrendered myself to the fact that I made it home. To this day, I still feel like I will always be taken care of here. It is a nice feeling. I am lucky. I can really use it now. I helped my mom prepare a dinner.

Before the afternoon ended, Jakoby and I were able to sneak out and go for a walk and play on the school playground. I enjoyed my time with him. We looked up at the old rock school building built in 1886. I reminisced about going to second grade there. I can still remember those creepy bathrooms in the basement with the rusty metal stalls and peeling red floors. I wouldn't use them. I would wait. I would wait too long and end up in a puddle somewhere on my way home from school.

Back on the playground, I carefully mapped out where the old monkey bars and the big metal slide had been. I carry a mark from those monkey bars to this day. On my first day of kindergarten, the boys were chasing the girls on the monkey bars. Soon, rocks and debris were flying, and it wasn't long before my forehead caught the brunt of the action. I remember the relief when I saw my mom's face through the big wooden door that day when she came to pick me up.

Jakoby tried every piece of equipment there. The kids today are so lucky with the tubes, climbing walls, and various whirligigs. Gone are those bolts and sharp metal edges, which caught every little knee. I am willing to bet a large percentage of middle-agers have one or two scars on the knees that can be attributed to a rusty screw on an old slide or merry-go-round.

I spun Jakoby on the merry-go-round and pushed him on the swings. We explored the slides together. It was the rope climb where I felt it again. It was a surge of determination and strength. I relished that moment. We took pictures, and I saved that feeling.

The next morning, Mom and I hung out and explored thrift stores. Afterwards, the perfect mocha was served up for me at the local coffee shop. I wrapped my hands around the nice steamy cup, perfect on that rainy day. In the foam, there was a heart-shaped design.

After lunch, we headed to my grandmother's house. It had been in a state of cleaning and sorting since her death three months ago. I was invited to come over today and sift through some clothing and jewelry to see if there was anything I wanted or needed.

The house still felt like my grandmother's even though much of the furniture had been moved out. The heart and soul were still there, some of the knickknacks and pictures, some family photos, still on the walls. I remember her showing off the colors of those walls hoping for her interior designer granddaughter's approval. I did not feel a sense of loss being in her home that day. I felt like she was still there.

Just three months ago, I sat beside her as she left us. She lay dying in that dark, little room, our shadows dancing on the wall behind her. As I held her arm, I felt her spirit, the energy between us, a warmth like no other. She was trying to tell me something. Although she could not speak, and I could not see the words she was dictating on an invisible notepad in the air, I seemed to understand what she was saying. It was reassurance all would be okay. I left with great peace. I lost my grandmother later that evening, but I had peace. I had peace with her death and everyone who had gone before her. I had peace with my own mortality and what a feeling that was.

As I rummaged through my grandmother's clothing and jewelry, I remembered her fondly. She took great pride in how she looked. I enjoyed hearing about the jewelry. Each piece had its own little history, where it came from, whom it came from. Some pieces were from family vacations, others from exotic locations, Mother's Day gifts.

My most cherished find of the day did not come from the jewelry drawer but from the kitchen utensils. I found my grandmother's melon baller. I have not owned a melon baller in years and have wanted to get one. I am a little tired of my chunky carelessly chopped fruit salad and long for one with consistent shapes. My grandmother made wonderful fruit salad (among many other things), which she lovingly brought to our family gatherings. I will enjoy making special fruit salads now.

I learned more about my grandmother that day. We found an old scrapbook containing pictures she drew back in 1925 when she was 9 years old. I knew she had artistic talents, ones that were most certainly passed to the next two generations that followed, but the scrapbook indicated that she truly had a gift. These drawings showed a young artist with a knack for perspective and portraits that were way beyond her years. Perhaps it was a gift never fully realized. It did reveal some insight into her interests and personality. What a wonderful gift for us to have these drawings to keep.

Later that afternoon, I took the kids to the Boscobel boat landing. I want the kids to experience my town, to describe to them a little bit about what my childhood was like. One special spot in Boscobel was the area by the bridge. I remember many a canoe trip ending here, where the swirling waters under the bridge turn into the quiet little boat landing. Across the river, the bluffs stand firmly. Between the bluffs are little valleys, each leading its way to little farms. Some families have lived here for generations in these valleys on their farms. The families change, the farms change, the bridge changes, but the river and the bluffs are permanent.

The sun is low in the sky as the day is drawing to a close. The boys are not enjoying the sunset view as much as I expected because the gnats have found us, and this time they are biting. I try to relax, take a deep breath, and enjoy the view. The boys climb the rocks down towards the water, but soon the gnats win, and we head back to the car.

On a whim I decide to cross the highway to an area to the east of the bridge. Here a gravel road and parking lot fronts the water and opens up to a lovely panorama of the bridge and the bluffs on the opposite side of the river. This is a favorite fishing spot for many. The boys ask if they can throw some rocks into the water here. I get out and join them, throwing a couple of rocks myself and following them down a little sand path that leads to the water. Looking back into the river bottoms, we could be in the middle of the Costa Rican rainforest. Overturned trees are intertwined with vines and had taken on a new life of their own. We find a little spot in the sand and begin drawing with sticks as water laps up to the shore. "I love you," I write. Next, we write, "Mom was here, Aleks was here, Jakoby was here."

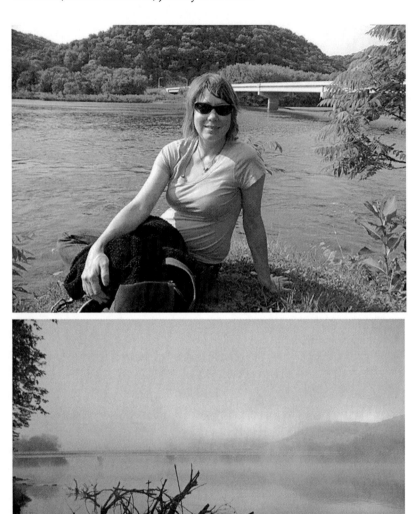

"Look!" Jakoby said as he gazed over the water. The sun had just broken through the clouds and cast a bright glow on the water. Above, the sun streaked through the clouds. It was beautiful.

Such a contrast on this side of the bridge—we were not bothered by the gnats, and it seemed we could stay here for hours exploring. Yes, the magic was there. I felt the difference.

The night is again filled with meals, laughter, family, and activity. Feeling the need for a break from the kids after two days of attention and closeness, I scheme a plan. The kids are planning to attend the morning movie at 10 a.m. There are a couple of places I need to visit again.

The morning arrives. Mom and Gary are departing this morning, so I will be alone with the kids. I urge them to move along quickly. There is at least one reluctant face, one that does not want to attend the movie. I do not accept this as an option as I start doling out the treat money.

The Blaine Theater in Boscobel has been around as long as I can remember. I walk into the entry and find that much has not changed on the inside either. The familiar smell of the buttery popcorn fills the air as a couple of high school students stand behind the small glass counter. The ticket prices have not changed much either. Today you can see a movie and have your popcorn and soda all for under $8. That's less than the ticket price where we come from. The kids are a little leery as I drop them in front of the theater. There is a sense of freedom being able to attend a movie on their own. I enjoy looking at the pile of bikes outside the theater. Ah, if all kids could do this.

I dash off to my first stop—the coffee shop. I decide not to get a mocha this time. This time I will enjoy a larger latte with two shots of espresso in a larger to-go cup. The woman has a friendly smile as she recognizes me from yesterday. I sit myself down and gaze around the shop at the green wainscoting, artwork from area schools, and posters for local benefits. A ceiling fan churns softly as the coffee brews. Next to me are some pot scrubbers and pot holders lovingly crocheted by local residents. A small can indicates that for a one- or two-dollar donation you can purchase one. One of the more colorful pot scrubbers catches my eye. I rummage through my purse and throw my last two dollars into the can, and soon I am off with my pot scrubber and latte.

My first stop is the cemetery. I don't go here too often when I come to town. It has been a long time since I have been up to see Dad. I will also go by Grandma and Grandpa's graves. It has been three months since Grandma's funeral. I pull in and park my car close to where I parked the day of the funeral. Grandma and Grandpa's graves are easy to find on the perimeter of the cemetery. I decide to walk from there up to find Dad. I have a general idea where he is, but I am not sure. It is a beautiful day. At 10 a.m. on this bright summer morning, the temperature is just right. The ground is still soft from the nighttime rains. The cemetery is full of mature trees, and in the morning the shadows cross my path as I walk from one section to the next. I enjoy the variety and the age of some of the grave markers. There are graves I recognize—an old teacher, a friend of my grandfather's. I walk for 15–20 minutes, and I still have not located Dad. I remember he was just to the south of one of the little roads that wind up and down the hillside cemetery. I decide it might be better to get my car. I will drive up and down the roads until I find it.

The Boscobel Cemetery is set on a hillside just above Kronshage Park. It is as old as the town itself with at least five generations buried there. The view from the higher parts of the cemetery are incredible, looking out to the bluffs that back up to the Wisconsin River. Depending on the time of year, you can look out to a sea of green or a dance of autumn colors.

Finally, I find it. Part of the problem is that a small bush had begun to obscure it. Under its shadow, the lichen and moss grew. I break a few branches of the bush and toss them away. The sunlight will prevent new growth of moss. I pick up a small stick and scratch away at the surface. I am not making much headway. I think for a moment of something I might have in my car to wipe it off. The pot scrubber would be perfect. I march over to my car and smile a little. It is if I feel a pull, something is guiding me. Soon I am down on my hands and knees scrubbing the surface. I feel the moisture from the ground soaking into my knees and onto my bare feet. With a small stick, I trace the engraved lines, "loving father of Stacey, Lauren, Garret, Lesley," until the words can be identified once again. I walk away satisfied.

I jump into my car and am determined to go back to the river spot that I visited with the boys yesterday. I need to go back just to make sure. I drive and finish my latte just before I get there. Today the parking lot has a couple of cars parked there. A family has just arrived and is preparing for a day of fishing. Two boys run to the shore and begin to throw rocks. There is something about this spot that just calls children to do that. Certainly, they will scare the fish away before they can even cast a line. I walk to the shore myself, passing two large stones that seem to mark an entry point.

The boys are about 30 feet to my right, and they call their father. They have just discovered something—bones, bones in the water. Their dad says it is a deer carcass. I take it as a symbol. I am not sure how a deer carcass got to this point, but here it laid and slowly made its way back into the water. A few feet in front of me is a deep channel. This is a strong river, this current swirling under the bridge and onward to the Mississippi and beyond.

The morning sun glazes the water. The skies are clear. Beyond the river, an eagle soars above one of the bluffs. I stare deep into the swirling waters in front of me. I sit on one of the rocks and close my eyes and breathe deeply. It is good to be alive. It is good to be present in this spot right now. If I should die, it is here that I would like to be laid to rest, not in the cemetery.

It is time to go. I walk calmly to my car and drive away from this spot. Back in town, I park my car and walk the streets of my former hometown, taking pictures all along the way. Timeless structures have withstood the test of time—the variety store, the creamery, the drugstore.

Soon the kids greet me and exit the movie theater. They are ready for their next big adventure, and I have a little more soul-searching to do. I gather them up, and we head out to Laurie's for swimming and lunch. I am greeted by my sister who looks relaxed and is wearing her swimsuit. I borrow a tank top for myself, and we find a nice sunny spot in the backyard and enjoy some conversation as the kids play in and around the pool. It is a perfect day to catch a few rays. We pop pizzas in the oven and serve some watermelon.

After lunch, the kids ask to go on an ATV ride. The boys will go first. While the boys are riding, Kassia and I play on the hillside. The light bounces off her shoulders as her beach cover-up flows with the breeze. I photograph her as the sunshine streams through the trees. There is something about the way she looks right now, still very childlike but her features just beginning to change. Soon she will be a beautiful young woman.

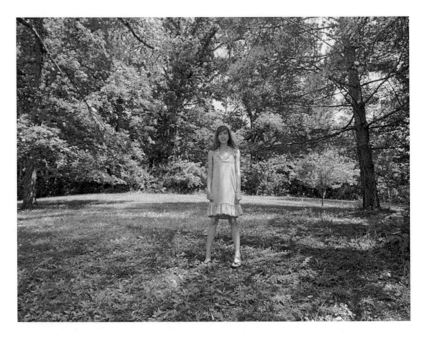

We are enjoying this moment in the sunshine among the trees. I am barefoot and feel the prickle underfoot of the sod. Some Shasta daisies are beginning to take root here and are bursting to the surface. I look around at this beautiful spot that is surrounded by nice solid oak trees. Two hawks are swirling around behind the house. I have found another spot.

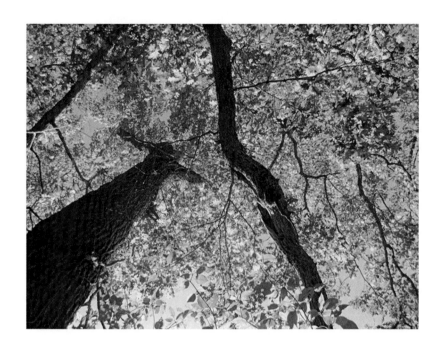

About the Authors

Carole Young is a retired art teacher and lives with her husband Gary and cat Sophie in a small town in the driftless area of SW Wisconsin. Her passion is her artwork and she especially loves doing portraits. She enjoys day trips with her book club friends, spending time with family and gardening.

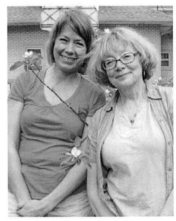

She is an admitted e-mail hoarder and that is what enabled her to assemble this book after her daughter's passing.

Mother's Day, 2011

Stacey Reynolds grew up in Boscobel Wisconsin. She graduated from the University of Wisconsin-Madison with a degree in interior design in 1986 and began working for Interior Systems, Inc. in Fond du Lac. During her career with ISI she designed the interiors of many McDonald's restaurants and Harley Davidson retail stores in the United States and abroad. She also studied architecture and urban planning at UW-Milwaukee.

She was married to Thomas M. Lesiewicz on the beach at Sandals in Ocho Rios, Jamaica, December 31, 1992, and they began their married life in Milwaukee. In 1994 they moved to Seattle, WA, where she continued to work for ISI for a time and then for The Environmental Home Center designing custom cabinets using eco-friendly materials. Their three children were born there.

They moved to Elgin, IL, in 2003 where she worked from home as an alternative energy consultant for Natural Dynamics, and volunteered her time at her children's pre-school (Elgin Parent Coop Preschool), elementary school (Lowrie PTA), her church (UUCE Green Sanctuary Committee), neighborhood community (SWAN-Southwest Area Neighbors), and in the larger Elgin community (Elgin Sustainability

Master Plan-Green Buildings and Technology). In 2009 she reached a life-long goal of receiving a black belt in Kyuki-do at Kim's Black Belt Academy in Elgin.

The Rise of Colon and Rectal Cancers in Young People

The above-titled article by Roni Caryn Rabin in the *New York Times* (February 28, 2017) cited a recent study done by the American Cancer Society that showed an increase in cancers of the colon and rectum in young people.

"Cancers of the colon and rectum have been declining in older adults in recent decades and have always been considered rare in young people. But scientists are reporting a sharp rise in colorectal cancers in adults as young as their 20s and 30s, an ominous trend," according to the story.

"The vast majority of colorectal cancers are still found in older people, with nearly 90 percent of all cases diagnosed in people over 50. But a new study from the American Cancer Society that analyzed cancer incidence by birth year found that colorectal cancer rates, which had dropped steadily for people born between 1890 and 1950, have been increasing for every generation born since 1950. Experts aren't sure why."

The study by the American Cancer Society concludes: Age-specific CRC risk has escalated back to the level of those born circa 1890 for contemporary birth cohorts, underscoring the need for increased awareness among clinicians and the general public, as well as etiologic research to elucidate causes for the trend. Further, as nearly one-third of rectal cancer patients are younger than age 55 years, screening initiation before age 50 years should be considered. (Colorectal Cancer Incidence Patterns in the United States, 1974–2013; Rebecca L. Siegel, Stacey A. Fedewa, William F. Anderson, Kimberly D. Miller, Jiemin Ma, Philip S. Rosenberg, Ahmedin Jemal; *Journal of the National Cancer Institute*, Volume 109, Issue 8, 1 August 2017, Published: 28 February 2017)